Operations Management in Radiology

ahra

ISBN: 978-0-9634176-5-7

Library of Congress Control Number: 2010904115

Orders and Customer Service: (800) 334-2472 or www.ahraonline.org

AHRA is the premier association for imaging professionals. Since 1973, the organization has led the industry in information, education, and professional support. Its programs–including its journal, *Radiology Management*; conferences; publications; and annual meeting–establish standards of excellence throughout the profession. In addition, AHRA's Certified Radiology Administrator (CRA) program is the first and only professional credential tailored specifically for radiology administrators. The CRA is designed to elevate professional standards, enhance individual performance, and recognize administrators who demonstrate knowledge essential to the practice of radiology management. The AHRA Education Foundation supports the membership and radiology professionals in the US and abroad by granting scholarships and conducting research that enhance the effectiveness of imaging and healthcare disciplines.

Contents

Acknowledgments

Operations Management in Radiology, the fifth book in the AHRA professional development series, came to fruition because of the hard work and relentless pursuit of a quality educational product by the many involved. We would like to show our appreciation to the following for their participation in the project.

Bayer HealthCare Pharmaceuticals continues to receive our gratitude and sincere appreciation for the generous grant which has made this development series possible. The time commitment and contributions of knowledge and expertise from the many authors and peer reviewers are much appreciated. The book would not have been possible without the input of each. The writing and editing skills contributed by Lynne Dodson brought every chapter of the project together as one final manuscript. The AHRA staff, under the direction of Debra L. Murphy, publications director, managed every aspect of the book from start to finish. From developing the outline and content of the material to finalizing the cover for print, Debra and her staff were there to make sure the project made it to the next step.

To everyone involved in this significant undertaking, we sincerely appreciate your efforts.

M. Shane Foreman, MSA
Laverna Hubbard, CRA
Luis O. Marquez, MBA, MPH, FAHRA, CRA

Bayer HealthCare
Pharmaceuticals

Introduction

Since the inception of the Certified Radiology Administrator (CRA) credential in 2002, AHRA: The Association for Medical Imaging Management, the preeminent organization for leaders in medical imaging management, has strived to develop educational materials specific to the field of imaging administration. Hence, the impetus for its professional development series of books. Along with its predecessors, *Financial Management in Radiology, Communication & Information Management in Radiology, Human Resource Management in Radiology,* and *Asset Management in Radiology, Operations Management in Radiology* continues the tradition of discussing material in depth to aid the continuing education of the imaging administrator.

The authors and reviewers of this book represent a cross section of today's imaging profession. Academic medical centers, community and rural hospitals, freestanding imaging centers, and private enterprise are represented among the contributors. This range of experience allows a broad perspective of ideas and expertise for the book material.

Operations Management in Radiology consists of four sections in which the building blocks and strategies of operations management are discussed:

Section 1, The Operational Foundation, reviews the baseline steps in developing the scope of service, building alliances, documenting processes, and developing procedures and protocols.

Section 2, Marketing Imaging Services, discusses the principles of marketing and specifically applies them to imaging facilities. Developing and evaluating a marketing program are also reviewed.

Section 3, Customer Management and Satisfaction, provides an overview of identifying the customer and targeting their needs (from patients to referring physicians). Satisfaction measurement tools, both qualitative and quantitative, are discussed, as well as methods for analyzing and applying selected data.

Section 4, Manage Performance Quality, reviews four commonly used improvement models and provides helpful examples and applications of these tools. Criteria are given for how to establish a quality improvement program that best meets your facility's needs.

This book addresses a wide variety of issues including documentation processes, alliance building, service strategy, customer management, marketing, and performance quality. Streamlined and strategic operations in the healthcare environment are fundamental contributors to organizational success. Managing these operations and their associated expenses, policies, and procedures requires expertise, know-how, and an acquired wisdom. *Operations Management in Radiology* is designed to provide the imaging administrator with the foundational knowledge in order to address these issues on a day-to-day and annual basis. This book is certain to become an important tool referenced time and again.

M. Shane Foreman, MSA
Laverna Hubbard, CRA
Luis O. Marquez, MBA, MPH, FAHRA, CRA

Editors

M. Shane Foreman, MSA

Principal & Founder

3D Health, Inc.

Chicago, Illinois

Shane helps establish and grow outpatient and physician businesses. He applies his 21 years of professional expertise and experience to working with hospitals, health systems, and physician group practices in defining and executing outpatient and medical staff strategies. Mr. Foreman has particular expertise in crafting niche imaging and medical staff strategies, growing and improving employed physician networks, and structuring hospital-physician joint ventures. Prior to founding 3d Health, Inc., Shane served as a director of the consultancy Tiber Group (now Navigant Consulting) in Chicago. He also served as regional director for Columbia (now HCA), vice president of business development for PhyServ, and chief financial officer with the Sisters of Charity of the Incarnate Word (now CHRISTUS). Shane has a BS in accounting from Louisiana College and an MSA in health services administration from Central Michigan University.

Laverna Hubbard, CRA

Executive Director

North State Radiology Medical Group

Chico, California

Laverna Hubbard has been the executive director for a 22 physician radiology group with over 100 employees in California for the past 15 years, serving 3 hospitals and 3 outpatient imaging centers. She is also the founder and president of Medical Business Solutions, a medical consulting company serving physicians and hospitals in California for over 18 years. Ms. Hubbard has over 30 years experience as an executive and entrepreneur in the successful development and management of imaging and medical practices. She has lectured for various organizations and published articles in several periodicals. She is a member of AHRA, RBMA, and MGMA and is also a Certified Radiology Administrator.

Luis O. Marquez, MBA, MPH, RT(R)(CT), CRA, FAHRA

Director of Imaging Services
The Methodist Hospitals, Inc.
Gary/Merrillville, Indiana

Luis O. Marquez is the director of imaging services for The Methodist Hospitals, Inc., a two-hospital system with an imaging center in northwest Indiana. Mr. Marquez has 12 years of senior radiology management experience in a wide range of healthcare facilities. He is an active member and Fellow of AHRA and a member of the American College of Healthcare Executives (ACHE). He graduated from Fort Hays State University with a bachelor of science in 1996. Luis went on to complete his master of public health from Wichita State University in 1998 and his MBA from Regis University in 2003. Mr. Marquez has served AHRA extensively by participating on the Annual Meeting Design Team, authoring articles in *Link* and *Radiology Management*, authoring chapters in the Professional Development Series books, presenting at the Annual Meeting, and hosting a Partners in Learning guest. He is a Certified Radiology Administrator.

Editor/Writer

J. Lynne Dodson

Creative Lines
Stratford, Connecticut

J. Lynne Dodson, a medical writer and editor since 1971, specializes in practice management, healthcare administration, patient education, and medical history. She is the author/co-author of 7 health-related books for general audiences, most recently, *Hot Times*, ghostwritten for bestselling nutritionist Ann Louise Gittleman, PhD. Ms. Dodson is also the author of 5 photographic histories of medicine and a contributing author to the *Journal of Oncology Practice*. She has twice won writing excellence awards from the American Medical Writers Association. Through her Stratford, CT based business, Creative Lines, she also provides public relations services to nonprofit organizations.

Contributors

Dana Allison, RT(R), BSM

Radiology Supervisor
Rady Children's Hospital San Diego
San Diego, California

Dana Allison is a supervisor for the radiology department at Rady Children's Hospital in San Diego, the only pediatric level 1 trauma center in the San Diego area. She returned to Rady's in January 2009, prior to that she was with Sharp Health Care in San Diego as a lead technologist for 6 years. She has been in the field of radiology for 20 years. Over the course of her career, Ms. Allison has spent much of her time working in pediatrics and is thrilled to be able to now bring her previous experience as a technologist to her leadership role. She earned her bachelor's degree in marketing in 2009. Ms. Allison has been an active member of the AHRA since joining in 2006 and has consistently served as an annual meeting volunteer and as a member of the 2010 Spring Conference Design Team.

Douglas Cathon, FAHRA

Director of Radiology and Imaging Services
Eden Medical Center
Castro Valley, California

Douglas has spent many years working up through the ranks, having worked in all modalities of imaging. He has been in imaging for over 40 years and an administrator for over 20 years, having had oversight of imaging facilities from a small 3 room, 6 staff operation to multiple hospitals to an academic center. Douglas has published over 40 articles and a book, *Management Dominos*, in 2006 and is an AHRA Fellow. His time, which includes many years in the military, has provided him with a deep understanding of how success is directly related to the people with whom we work.

Ernesto A. Cerdena, CRA, MS, RT(R)(CT)(CV), FACHE

Operations Manager of Ambulatory Imaging Services
Assistant Director of Radiology
Stamford Hospital
Stamford, Connecticut

Ernie Cerdena is the operations manager of ambulatory imaging services and assistant director of radiology at Stamford Hospital in Stamford, CT. He holds a master's degree in organizational leadership from Mercy College in New York and is pursuing his PhD in healthcare/business administration. He is a CRA and a Fellow by the American College of Healthcare Executives. He has volunteered in many capacities for AHRA, including as Annual Meeting Design Team chair, an author for *Radiology Management* and a member of its Editorial Review Board, and a director on the Education Foundation Board.

Richard Egan, CRA, MBA, MS
Administrative Director of Medical Imaging
Haywood Regional Medical Center
Clyde, North Carolina
Rich Egan has been in the radiology business for over 25 years. He joined Haywood Regional Medical Center in Clyde, NC as Administrative Director of Medical Imaging in 2008. He manages both the medical imaging department as well as the cardiac catheterization lab. Rich is an active member of AHRA and is a CRA. Interestingly, he has performed radiographic procedures for the Miami Dolphins (NFL), Miami Heat (NBA) and the Florida Panthers (NHL).

Janice Eurton, CRA, RT(R)(M)
Manager Out Patient Imaging
Clark Memorial Hospital
Jeffersonville, Indiana
Janice Eurton is the manager of a hospital owned outpatient imaging center for Clark Memorial Hospital. She holds a master's degree in management and leadership from Webster University and has over 35 years of experience in the field of imaging, with the last 15 years serving in a management role. Ms. Eurton is an active member of the AHRA, obtaining her CRA in 2006, serving as Design Team chair of the 2007 Fall Conference and as a Design Team member of the 2009 and 2010 Annual Meetings. She also sits on the Editorial Review Board for *Radiology Management*, is a speaker for AHRA, and has published various imaging articles. In addition, Ms. Eurton is a member of the American Society of Radiologic Technologists.

Barbara A. Hubley, MPAH
Director, Clinical Support Services
Massachusetts General Hospital
Boston, Massachusetts
Barbara Hubley has been employed at Massachusetts General Hospital for close to 20 years. The last 12 years she has been in the role of director of clinical support

services in the imaging department. Her leadership responsibilities have included scheduling, image management, nursing, engineering, and customer service. As a senior consultant for the Radiology Consultant Group, she has consulted nationally and internationally on a variety of topics related to healthcare delivery systems. She holds a master's degree in public administration in healthcare from Suffolk University in Boston, MA.

Robert E. Jacoby, BBA, CRA, RT(R)
Administrative Director Radiology
Pomona Valley Hospital Medical Center
Pomona, California
Robert Jacoby has held the position of administrative director of radiology at Pomona Valley Hospital Medical Center in Pomona, CA for the past 12 years. He has held previous leadership positions at other hospitals and outpatient based facilities throughout southern California. Mr. Jacoby has served the AHRA in a variety of capacities, such as participating as a Design Team member, authoring articles in *Link* and *Radiology Management*, lecturing at the Annual Meeting, acting as team leader for the *Compensation & Benefits Survey*, and hosting a coding seminar and Partners in Learning guest. He holds a bachelors degree in business administration and is also a Certified Radiology Administrator.

Jennifer Kroken, MBA
Revenue Cycle Consultant
Healthcare Resource Providers
Dallas, Texas
Jennifer Kroken is a consultant with Healthcare Resource Providers based in Albuquerque, NM. She has been a healthcare consultant for 9 years and also acts as operations manager for Radiology Consultants of North Dallas in Dallas, TX. Prior to joining HRP, she worked for 8 years in various radiology billing and administrative capacities in Albuquerque, NM. She has presented at national conferences for the RBMA and has been published in several industry publications.

Kathy Tabor McEwan
Executive Director
Boca Raton Community Hospital
Boca Raton, Florida
Kathy Tabor McEwan held various management and leadership positions at Massachusetts General Hospital in Boston, MA prior to becoming the executive director of imaging at Boca Raton Community Hospital. Her technical background

includes work in MRI, CT, interventional, radiation therapy planning, emergency radiology, and contrast media research. She has consulted nationally and internationally, published a variety of articles and abstracts, and has been a guest lecturer at national and international conferences. She is a senior consultant with RCG Healthcare and has significant experience in workflow management, project planning, and tactical project implementation. She holds a bachelor's degree from Harvard University in Cambridge, MA.

Suzanne Ramthun, RT(R), MBA, CRA, CIIP
Radiology Director
Assistant Professor of Radiology
Mayo Clinic College of Medicine
Rochester, Minnesota
Sue Ramthun is a radiology director at Mayo Clinic Rochester. She has worked in Mayo Radiology for 36 years and the past 12 years in the director role with oversight of electronic imaging and the campus filmless conversion. Ms. Ramthun has been an AHRA member since 1990 and a member of the Society for Imaging Informatics in Medicine (SIIM) since 2000. In 2007 she passed the CRA and in 2009 became an American Board of Imaging Informatics Certified Imaging Informatics Professional (CIIP).

Philip L. Ruth, MBA, RT(R)
Director of Medical Imaging and Radiation Therapy
St Joseph's Mercy Health Center
Hot Springs, Arkansas
Philip Ruth is the director of medical imaging and radiation therapy at St. Joseph's Mercy Health System in Hot Springs, AR. St Joseph's is a 315 bed, level 2 trauma center. He has been involved in the imaging field since 1975 in various capacities and an imaging administrator for over 24 years. He received his bachelor of science and master's of business administration in healthcare management from Century University in Albuquerque, NM. He has been an active member of AHRA since 1993 and is currently serving on the *Radiology Management* Editorial Review Board. Philip has also written for the journal, as well as AHRA's newsletter, *Link*.

Sue Rysted
Assistant Coordinator
Mayo Clinic Rochester
Rochester, Minnesota
Sue Rysted is the assistant coordinator to the radiology asset manager at Mayo Clinic Rochester. She has worked in Mayo radiology for 27 years in various

management and technologist roles. Ms. Rysted obtained her MRI certification in 1995 and CRA certification in 2007. She completed her bachelor's degree in health arts in 2005 and master's of business administration in 2009, both through the St. Francis University at Joliet, IL. She has been a member of the AHRA since 2006, having been involved in volunteer opportunities including serving on the 2009 and 2010 webinar design teams.

Bonni J. Standley, FACHE, FAHRA, CRA, MBA, BSRT(R)(MR)
Director of Radiology
Mayo Clinic
Rochester, Minnesota
Bonni is the director of radiology where she serves the practice and education divisions at the Mayo Clinic of Rochester, MN. Mayo Clinic Rochester has 1950+ beds and 1200 FTEs in imaging. She has worked in radiology for 25 years. Bonni holds master's degrees in business and healthcare administration and a bachelor of science in radiology. She is an active member of AHRA, ACHE, and the ASRT. Bonni has served AHRA for two terms on the board of directors and is currently on the executive board. She has served three years on the Strategic Planning Committee, was chair of the 2009 Minnesota regional meeting, Radiology Administration Certification Commission (RACC) CRA exam rewrite committee, and other various volunteer activities for AHRA. Bonni is a frequent presenter for the Leadership Institute.

Kathy Williams, RT(R)(CT), CRA, MA
Radiology Supervisor
Mayo Clinic Rochester
Rochester, Minnesota
Kathy Williams is a radiology supervisor at Mayo Clinic Rochester. She has 12 years of experience in supervisory roles and is involved with various radiology projects that are interesting and challenging. In 2008 Ms. Williams passed the CRA and in 2009 she graduated from St. Mary's University with a master's of arts degree in management.

Reviewers

Tonya Bell Brightmon, MS
Mgr. Diagnostic Imaging—
Interventional Radiology
MD Anderson Cancer Center
Houston, Texas

Debbie Clark
Assistant Director of Imaging
Erie County Medical Center
Buffalo, New York

Joseph R. Dilone, CIIP, CPAS, LMRT, ARMRIT
Radiology Administrator, PACS
Administrator
Texas Medical Management Services
Houston, Texas

Gabriel Dreiling
Practice Manager
Valley Imaging Center
Athens, Alabama

Gina M. Greenwood, MBA
Radiology Business Operations Manager
University of Wisconsin Hospital
Madison, Wisconsin

Donald E. Hatley, Jr.
Administrative Supervisor
Armed Forces Institute of Pathology
Alexandria, Virginia

Lynn Imel, BS, RT(R)(M), RVT
Administrative Director of Radiology
Marion General Hospital
Marion, Indiana

Joe Larson, CRA
Medical Imaging Manager
Multicare Health System
Tacoma, Washington

Kirk Lawson
Administrative Director Radiology
NYU Medical Center
New York, New York

Angelic P. McDonald, MS
CT/MR Manager
Cypress-Fairbanks Medical Center
Houston, Texas

Judy Offenback
Radiology Manager
Virginia Physicians, Inc
Glen Allen, Virginia

Peggy A. Pust, CRA
Director of Imaging Services
Monongalia General Hospital
Morgantown, West Virginia

Jason Scott, MBA, RT(R)(MR)
Chief Technologist, MRI/CT
St. Elizabeth Regional Health
Lafayette, Indiana

Eileen Stearman, CRA
Radiology Manager
Christus St. Michael Health System
Texarkana, Texas

Leland Taylor, MBA, RT(R)
Director of Radiology
Vaughan Regional Medical Center
Selma, Alabama

Jason C. Theadore, MHA, CRA, RT(R)
Director of Diagnostic and Therapeutic Services
OhioHealth
Columbus, Ohio

Pamela Sue Wickkiser, MBA
Radiology Manager
Humboldt General Hospital
Winnemucca, Nevada

1 The Operational Foundation

In this section:

- Chapter 1: Develop the Scope of Service
- Chapter 2: Build Alliances
- Chapter 3: Document Processes to Ensure Service Delivery
- Chapter 4: Develop Examination Protocols and Evaluate Results

Chapter 1

Develop the Scope of Service

Dana Allison

Medical researchers continually find new ways to use radiation and other imaging technologies. The state of the art industry challenges imaging professionals to establish and maintain a scope of service that both meets the needs of customers and remains within fiscal constraints. These services should be reassessed frequently based on changes in customer needs, government regulations, reimbursement policies, and imaging technology.

Scope of service is the framework that defines a business and provides the structure for developing a business plan and/or strategy. By informing internal and external parties about services and capabilities, it sets clear expectations. Imaging staff, the organization as a whole, healthcare providers, the community, and patients benefit the most.

At the least, scope of service defines:

- Mission and/or vision
- Services and capabilities
- Hours of operation and locations (if multifacility)
- Patient population
- Staffing plan or model
- Competencies and professional standards

The scope of service may also impact facility accreditations; technologies used such as the choice of analog or digital instrumentation, a picture archiving and communication system (PACS), electronic medical records (EMRs), and aseptic techniques; and criteria governing admissions, transfers, and discharges.

An imaging facility's scope of service can be defined by its degree of differentiation. At the most basic level, all facilities offer:

- Reception and scheduling
- Diagnostic and therapeutic procedures
- Transcription and report distribution

- Film filing, digital imaging processing, and image distribution
- Clinical consultations
- Financial consultations (payment arrangements)

Within the categories of diagnostic and therapeutic imaging, a focus on one or more subspecialties further expands the scope of service. These subspecialties include:

- General X-ray and fluoroscopy
- Nuclear medicine
- Magnetic resonance imaging (MRI)
- Computed tomography (CT)
- Ultrasound
- Interventional radiology (angiography)
- Positron emission testing (PET)
- Mammography

Each subspecialty presents a wide range of examinations from which to choose. For example, Sidebar 1.1 offers a possible list of nuclear medicine procedures.

Within a hospital, one or more of these subspecialties may be offered in the imaging department, the emergency department, or even at the patient's bedside. Services may be available on either an inpatient or outpatient basis.

A number of factors will influence the selection of services that will constitute a facility's scope, including the organization's size, the availability of expertise, the

SIDEBAR 1.1: Examinations Within the Subspecialty of Nuclear Medicine

Bone marrow scan
Bone scan
Brain scan
Brain single photon emission computed tomography (SPECT)
Cisternogram
Gallium imaging
Gastric emptying scan
Gastrointestinal bleed scan
Hepatobiliary scan
Hepatobiliary scan with ejection fraction
Liver/spleen scan
Lung perfusion/ventilation scan
Lung quantification scan
Lymphoscintigraphy
Meckel's diverticulum scan
Multigated acquisition scan (MUGA)
Myocardial infarction coronarography
Myocardial perfusion SPECT
Octreoscan
Parathyroid scan
Radioactive iodine therapy
Renal scan
Thyroid cancer whole body scan
Thyroid uptake scan

Box 1.1 Scope of Service Template

Scope of Services	Last Reviewed/Revised Date:	No. of Pages:
	X	X
Care Area/Department/ Unit Name	Point of Contact:	Telephone Number:
	X	X

1. **Description of Program/Service:**
2. **Patient Population Served:**

   Age Criteria:
   Common Diagnoses:
   Common Treatments/Procedures/Activities:
   Important Aspects of Care:
   Admission, Transfer, and Discharge Criteria:

3. **Location of Program and Hours of Operation:**
4. **Staffing Plan:**
5. **Competencies for Each Position:**
6. **Professional Standards:**

financial climate internal and external to the facility, and its customer base and/or markets. These factors are closely interrelated. Changes in one will almost always necessitate changes in one or more of the others and may also require changes in the scope of service. See Box 1.1 for a sample scope of service template.

Facility Size as a Factor in Service Selection

An imaging unit within a major university hospital is likely to have a broader scope of service than one within a small community hospital or a freestanding center in a rural community. University hospitals take part in clinical studies of new technologies and new applications of existing technology. Furthermore, as training facilities for new physicians, these hospitals must provide opportunities to learn about the wide range of procedures and devices the physicians will encounter in their practices. Access to sophisticated, leading-edge technology also helps attract top tier faculty physicians and researchers, who in turn bring grant dollars to help fund further service offerings.

A facility's physical size can also limit its access to imaging technology, given the special space requirements many imaging devices demand. For example, a vendor's template for installation of an MRI scanner may call for 600 sq ft for the scanner. However, the necessary space is closer to 1700 sq ft when a control room, equipment room, patient areas, and even the substantial walls needed for MRI operation are included.

Size factors such as these must be taken into consideration in defining the facility's service offerings. Attempting to provide services without the appropriate organizational or physical size is likely to lead to increased employee stress, low staff morale, and poor customer service. When pressure mounts from customers or staff radiologists to expand or change the scope of service, management faced with size limitations must explore a range of options. In the example of an MRI, these options include leasing a portable MRI, buying a competitor's facility, negotiating an alliance with another practice, renovating existing space, or building a new facility.

Expertise as a Factor in Service Selection

An organization should not attempt to offer a service without adequate staff qualified to perform that service. If a facility adds an interventional radiologist to its staff, for example, it must ensure that certified and trained personnel (eg, an interventional imaging nurse) are also on staff before interventional services can be offered. In such cases, a list of every employee's certifications, licenses, skills, and training, updated regularly, can be a valuable resource in planning changes to the service offerings.

Rural or community-based facilities may have difficulty attracting imaging subspecialists, thereby potentially limiting the scope of service. In the early years of an effective new procedure or technology, for example, few physicians and even fewer support staff will be qualified. The competition for those who are will be fierce. As more subspecialists complete the necessary training and certification, facilities in less desirable communities may still face stiff competition for these subspecialists. To offer such services, it may be necessary to share a subspecialist with a nearby medical school, tertiary hospital, or community-based center. In some instances, teleradiology may allow specialists to remotely carry out examinations or consultations.

Finances as a Factor in Service Selection

The financial climate affects all aspects of modern healthcare, including what services can and will be available. Internally, a facility with a strong balance sheet and access to capital has the financial capability to invest in equipment, space, and personnel. This ensures maximum flexibility in terms of the services that can be offered. Providing services that meet the needs of patients and are adequately reimbursed, in turn, strengthens the balance sheet.

On the other hand, external forces can be a powerful influence. Most notably, when Medicare and private insurers reimburse at a level significantly below cost or refuse to pay for a procedure, the decision to offer that procedure must be analyzed. Will the procedure make such a significant difference to a group of patients that the financial considerations become secondary, at least for the present? Should the procedure be provided to those able to pay with the hope that as its effectiveness is more powerfully demonstrated, the insurers will change their policy? Can the practice take part in a clinical trial that will reimburse the practice to make the procedure available to patients who benefit from it?

Other external actions with the potential to financially affect a facility's service offerings include changes at the local, state, and federal levels in business taxes and regulations, which increase the costs of providing one or more services.

The Market as a Factor in Service Selection

Unlike some healthcare services (eg, heart transplants), imaging services are typically local—patients seldom travel great distances for a chest X-ray, and physicians seldom build referral networks with distant radiologists. Thus, when a facility determines its scope of service, it must examine the needs of customers, the demographics of the community, and the trends in the local healthcare market.

Offering services that the majority of customers want and need is the basis for any successful healthcare facility. With a heavy reliance on physician referrals, an imaging practice must remain open to suggestions from not only patients but also their physicians. Customer satisfaction surveys, focus groups, and face-to-face meetings are useful tools to remain in touch with patient and physician imaging needs.

Beyond the current customer base, the demographics for the community at large should be considered. An imaging facility in a ski community, for example, might find its general radiography and MRI services in great demand, but may not be able to justify adding PET for mammography to its scope of service. In reviewing demographics as an indicator of needed services, issues such as growth rate (eg, births, deaths, immigration, emigration), average age (eg, Medicare population, pediatric population), and socioeconomics (eg, average household income, level of education) should be considered.

No decisions about an imaging facility's scope of services should be made without considering the other imaging providers in the community and trends in the community's healthcare market in general. In many markets today, providers include not just hospital-based imaging departments and freestanding imaging centers, but also other medical specialties (eg, cardiologists offering CT angiography or orthopedists with their own MRI). Issues such as the following should be tracked:

- Pending health legislation at the local, state, and national level
- Changes in service offerings at competitive facilities
- The introduction of new healthcare facilities within the market
- The availability of trained, certified staff in the local job market

From a broader market perspective, technologists and other staff members should be encouraged to bring news of developments within their field to management's attention (eg, new ways existing technology is being used or recommendations by professional associations about certifications).

Identify Regulatory Standards

Determining an imaging facility's scope of service must be done within a context of myriad standards and regulations governing everything from worker protection to patient privacy. Both government agencies and nongovernmental organizations are responsible for interpreting the governing documents, providing information and training to aid implementation, and monitoring facilities to ensure compliance. No additions, deletions, or changes to services should be made without reviewing the relevant regulations from the following agencies and organizations (presented in alphabetical order).

American College of Radiology

The American College of Radiology (ACR) is a professional society comprised of 32,000 members, primarily radiologists, radiation oncologists, clinical medical physicists, interventional radiologists, and nuclear medicine physicians. Founded in 1923, it aims to encourage continuing education, improve radiologic services to patients, and advance the field.

Among the ways the ACR accomplishes its goals is to issue technical standards and practice guidelines in the areas of general diagnostic radiology, breast imaging, interventional radiology, medical physics, nuclear medicine, radiologic oncology, and ultrasound. These documents are not intended as requirements of practice, but as educational tools to aid in providing effective and safe medical care in the imaging setting (Sidebar 1.2).

SIDEBAR 1.2: Topics Covered by the ACR Technical Standard for Diagnostic Procedures Using Radiopharmaceuticals

Definition

Qualifications of personnel

A. Physician
B. Nuclear medicine technologist
C. Qualified medical physicist or other qualified scientist

Radiopharmacy

A. Responsibility
B. Radiopharmaceuticals
C. Elution of generators and onsite preparation of radiopharmaceutical "kits"
D. Records

Instrument quality control

A. For all scintillation cameras
B. For single photon emission computed tomography (SPECT)
C. For Xenon or DTPA Aerosol delivery system
D. Hard-copy imaging device
E. Film processors
F. Geiger counters, well counters, ionization chambers
G. Radionuclide dose calibrators
H. Daily instrument notes

Patient and personnel safety

Procedure manual

Records

Radiation safety in imaging

Quality control and improvement, safety, infection control, and patient education concerns

Abbreviation: ACR, American College of Radiology.

Source: Adapted from *Practice Guidelines and Technical Standards*. Reston, VA: American College of Radiology; 2008:1203–1209. Available at: http://www.acr.org/SecondaryMainMenuCategories/quality_safety/guidelines/nuc_med/radiopharmaceuticals.aspx. Accessed July 14, 2009.

In addition, the US Food and Drug Administration (FDA) has designated the ACR as an accrediting body for all facilities offering mammography services. Accreditation is a prerequisite for certification under the Mammography Quality Standards Act (MQSA) regulations, with which every mammography unit must comply.

Department of Health and Human Services

The Centers for Medicare & Medicaid Services (CMS) is a federal agency within the US Department of Health and Human Services (HHS) that is currently responsible for administering the Medicare and Medicaid programs. CMS also oversees compliance with the regulations of the Health Insurance Portability and Accountability Act (HIPAA) in conjunction with the Office for Civil Rights within the same department.

Enacted in 1996, HIPAA was intended to improve individuals' ability to transfer health insurance coverage from one employer to another and to encourage conversion by the healthcare industry to electronic medical recordkeeping. However, growing concerns over privacy of health information and security of electronic records led Congress to broaden the legislation's provisions. When planning or revising a facility's scope of service, the Privacy and Security Rules need to be addressed, especially if alliances with other parties are being considered to provide the service.

The Privacy Rule

The Privacy Rule covers all individually identifiable health information (referred to as protected health information [PHI]) used or disclosed by the department or facility (eg, ultrasound examination results, radiographic images bearing patient identification). The privacy provisions apply to all forms of PHI, including oral comments, paper documents, or electronic files. The rule's provisions seek to (a) give patients access to and control over the use of their medical records; (b) restrict use of a patient's PHI to direct healthcare purposes, while recognizing legitimate needs for medical research and public health; and (c) maintain PHI security. Among the key requirements, every healthcare facility must develop procedures designed to[1]:

- Restrict PHI access to the minimum necessary to ensure quality care
- Verify the identity of people asking for PHI
- Obtain patient consent and authorization to disclose or use PHI
- Educate patients about their rights to privacy
- Safeguard the intentional or accidental disclosure of PHI
- Train personnel in privacy procedures

The Office for Civil Rights, which is responsible for enforcing the Privacy Rule, seeks to voluntarily achieve compliance but will investigate facilities through complaints or reports of lost health data filed with the office or by random compliance reviews. In 2008, over 8500 complaints were received.[2] If the investigators determine a failure to comply was deliberate or was not promptly corrected, monetary penalties up to $50,000 per violation can be imposed. In addition, individuals who knowingly obtain or disclose PHI can face criminal penalties including fines and imprisonment.[1]

The Security Rule

The Security Rule, enforced by the CMS, focuses on ensuring the confidentiality, integrity, and availability of electronic medical records. Like the Privacy Rule, the Security Rule requires health facilities to devise safeguards in three categories: administrative (eg, training, contingency planning), physical (eg, workstation use, laptop security), and technical (eg, password protection, data encryption). Unlike the Privacy Rule, however, the Security Rule provides a much more comprehensive and detailed set of security requirements, which are nevertheless technology neutral and adaptable for the size and level of risk of a facility.

Any facility that has access to PHI electronically should carry out the following process to ensure compliance[3]:

1. Assess current security, risks, and gaps.
2. Develop an implementation plan.
3. Implement security measures and solutions that are reasonable and appropriate.
4. Document all security decisions, including the analysis, rationale, and final decision, especially as they relate to those specifications in the rule that are not "required" (referred to as "addressable implementation specifications").
5. Reassess security measures periodically. In particular, before implementing a new service or changing an existing one, security measures should be reviewed in place for modifications needed to accommodate the changing scope of service.
6. Confirm all informatics systems have a disaster recovery plan in place.

The procedures, process, and penalties to ensure compliance of the Security Rule are similar to those for the Privacy Rule. Whenever possible, voluntary compliance is sought, but fines, requirements for community service or repeated security audits, and criminal prosecution can be applied for willful failure to meet standards.

Food and Drug Administration

An agency of the US federal government, the Food and Drug Administration (FDA) is responsible for protecting public health by ensuring that safe and effective products reach the market and by monitoring those products for continued safety once they are in use. Through the Center for Devices and Radiological Health, the agency issues standards for CT, mammography, fluoroscopy, and medical X-rays. Generally, these standards have a direct impact on device manufacturers, who must ensure that their devices meet or exceed the FDA requirements before being sold. However, as imaging facilities are the end users, they are subject to FDA issued recall notices for installed equipment.

As noted above, to operate legally, facilities offering mammography services must be certified under the MQSA program, which is administered and enforced by the FDA. The MQSA, enacted in 1992 with final regulations effective in 1999, seeks to ensure the quality of mammography nationwide. The legislation contains 3 sections. The first specifies the process by which agencies can become accreditation bodies and their responsibilities. In 2009 the ACR and the states of Arkansas, Iowa, and Texas were FDA approved accreditation bodies. The second section describes the role of imaging facilities in being accredited and certified. The third section details the requirements for state agencies that seek to become FDA approved certification agencies, which in 2009 were the states of Illinois, Iowa, South Carolina, and Texas.[4] Any state can enact stricter legislation than the MQSA, and all states work with the FDA to ensure the federal regulations are enforced.

The second section of the MQSA is particularly relevant, as it specifies the activities imaging facilities must carry out to receive and maintain accreditation and certification. These cover the following areas:

- Qualifications of interpreting physicians, imaging technologists, and medical physicists working for the facility
- Requirements for mammography equipment, ranging from minimum specifications for image receptor sizes to the types of compression available
- Results reporting, medical records, and patient access to information
- Quality assurance requirements, including an organized program of regular quality control tests to be carried out on equipment by a quality control technologist and/or a medical physicist; a medical outcomes audit program to follow up positive mammogram results; a patient complaint mechanism; and a clinical image quality review program

Facilities must carry out and report the results of an annual survey conducted by a medical physicist, as well as be subject to inspection at least once every 3 years or whenever a reason to suspect problems arises. Those who fail to maintain standards are subject to monetary fines, community service requirements, and suspension or revocation of accreditation and/or certification. If a review of images finds their poor quality represents a serious risk to human health, the facility can be required to notify all affected patients and their referring physicians. Professionals can lose their positions and license to practice mammography.

Each year, the FDA issues a report summarizing actions taken against facilities and the outcomes. In addition, it maintains a list of all MQSA certified facilities in the US, accessible to patients and their physicians on their Web site. A total of 8817 facilities were fully MQSA certified as of December 2008.[4]

The Joint Commission

The Joint Commission is a nongovernmental, not-for-profit organization that aims to improve the quality of healthcare by providing accreditation and related services nationwide. Founded in 1951 by representatives of the American Hospital Association, American Medical Association, American College of Physicians, and American College of Surgeons, The Joint Commission originally focused on the voluntary accreditation of hospitals. While it continues to accredit hospitals, including their imaging departments, in 1975 the organization developed the Ambulatory Health Care accreditation program, which applies to freestanding diagnostic imaging centers, mobile imaging units, and imaging practices, among other ambulatory practices.

While accreditation theoretically remains voluntary, more than 30 states recognize the commission's accreditation as fulfilling some or all regulatory requirements.[5] In addition, many managed care contractors, third-party payers, and regulatory agencies require the commission's accreditation for reimbursement or certification (eg, CMS accepts accreditation in granting Medicare certification). Accreditation may also improve access to or lower the cost of liability insurance coverage.[5]

The process of achieving and maintaining accreditation relies on onsite surveys by trained reviewers, unannounced once initial accreditation is achieved (Sidebar 1.3). The surveys now focus on National Patient Safety Goals (Sidebar 1.4) and use what is referred to as tracer methodology. The reviewers randomly select patient charts and retrace the patient's steps through each unit, asking the staff questions and reviewing procedures along the way. A report is issued, providing guidance on areas that fail to meet standards. Organizations that meet standards or correct failures to subsequently meet standards are accredited for 3 years.

In an accredited facility, any new services or changes to existing ones must conform to the commission's standards and goals. Opportunities for new services may also arise from efforts to meet the goals. For example, one safety goal is to ensure timely reporting of critical results. A mammography center could offer a new service that provides "results while you wait" and a consultation with a radiologist for women with positive results following a screening mammography.

National Committee for Quality Assurance

Founded in 1990, the National Committee for Quality Assurance (NCQA) is a not-for-profit organization focused on improving healthcare quality, especially

SIDEBAR 1.3: Sample Agenda for an Initial Survey by The Joint Commission

Day 1 (8 AM to 4:30 PM)

Opening Conference

Introductions

Surveyor planning needs (requested by Surveyor for Planning Session)

- List of active patients (by service) with name, address, and diagnosis/procedure
- Priority Focus Process
- High-level organization chart
- List of departments/units/areas/programs/services within the organization (if applicable)
- Key contact person who can assist surveys in planning tracer selection
- List of eligible contracts (direct services)
- Environment of care management plans
- Environment of care multidisciplinary team meeting minutes for past 12 months
- Performance improvement data
- Measures of Success data from previous Periodic Performance Review (resurveys only)
- Infection control data

Orientation to healthcare organization

- A high-level orientation to the organization (vision, mission, community, etc)

Surveyor Planning Session

- Review the Priority Focus Process information
- Review Measures of Success (when applicable)
- Review list of eligible contracts
- Review list of current patients
- Quick overview of performance improvement and infection control data
- Select patients for Tracer Methodology
- Finalize agenda activities

Individual Care Tracer Activity

Tracers may include:

- Review of closed clinical records
- Patient/family member interview
- Site visits
- Pharmacy visit (as applicable)
- Patient care areas (ie, ambulatory infusion, examination room)
- Interdisciplinary team interview

Lunch

Individual Care Tracer Activity continued

Survey Team Meeting/Planning Session

Leadership Session

- Discussion of critical systems analysis exploration—leadership probes on some of the critical processes
- Discussion of organization-wide performance improvement activities as appropriate to type and scope of services

Special Issue Resolution

Day 2 (8 AM to 4:30 PM)

Daily Briefing

Systems Tracer

- Discussion with appropriate staff regarding the use of data for improvement purposes, and the management of medical and infection control issues

Individual Care Tracer Activity

Environment of Care Session

- Review of management plans
- Review evaluation of emergency plan
- Review system for reporting accidents, injuries, and safety hazards; identification of any trends; implementing and monitoring of improvement
- Building tour for Life Safety Code compliance (if applicable)

Lunch

Human Resources/Credentials Review

- Selected records to include healthcare professionals of interest pertaining to Tracer activities
- Includes contract staff

Surveyor Report Preparation

CEO Exit Briefing and Organization Exit Conference

Source: Adapted from *Ambulatory Care Accreditation Handbook*. Oak Terrace, IL: Joint Commission on Accreditation of Healthcare Organizations; 2009:29–30.

among health plans and their providers. Its certification and accreditation programs are voluntary and involve both offsite and onsite evaluations on as many as 60 standards and 40 areas of performance. Organizations that achieve certification or accreditation are listed on the NCQA Web site, available for review and comparison by potential patients. Health plans who achieve accreditation are exempt from many or all aspects of annual state audits in more than 30 states; failure to achieve accreditation may mean the health plan will not be available to employees of many major corporations.[6]

Among the organization's credentials is the Physician Organization Certification Program, available to single specialty or multispecialty practices. The program's

SIDEBAR 1.4: The Joint Commission National Patient Safety Goals

Goal 1. Improve the accuracy of patient identification.
Goal 2. Improve the effectiveness of communication among caregivers.
Goal 3. Improve the safety of using medications.
Goals 4 to 6. Retired.
Goal 7. Reduce the risk of healthcare-associated infections.
Goal 8. Accurately and completely reconcile medications across the continuum of care.
Goal 9. Reduce the risk of patient harm resulting from falls.
Goal 10. Reduce the risk of influenza and pneumococcal disease in institutionalized older adults.
Goal 11. Reduce the risk of surgical fires.
Goal 12. Not applicable.
Goal 13. Encourage patients' active involvement in their own care as a patient safety strategy.
Goal 14. Prevent healthcare-associated pressure ulcers (decubitus ulcers).
Goal 15. The organization identifies safety risks inherent in its patient population.
Goal 16. Improve recognition and response to changes in a patient's condition.

Source: Adapted from The Joint Commission on Accreditation of Healthcare Organizations. 2010 National patient safety goals. http://www.jointcommission.org/PatientSafety/NationalPatientSafetyGoals. Accessed January 15, 2010.

Quality Management and Improvement category, for example, evaluates a range of quality improvement activities including:

- The presence of a quality improvement committee that meets regularly and works under an annual work plan
- The collection of practice safety and quality data, which is made available to staff and patients
- Regular review of customer satisfaction, with actions to improve performance based on comments
- The use of regularly reviewed practice guidelines against which to measure performance

Even if a facility does not wish to apply for certification on its own behalf, it may be measured by health plans and other insurers using NCQA's standardized measurement tool, the Healthcare Effectiveness Data and Information Set (HEDIS). According to NCQA, more than 90% of US health plans use HEDIS to measure performance on care and service of plan providers.[6] Of particular note to imaging facilities are the HEDIS measures on breast cancer screening. Failure to achieve performance levels may lead to loss of contracts; those with NCQA certification or accreditation may lose their status and be dropped from the organization's Web-based report card.

Nuclear Regulatory Commission

The US Nuclear Regulatory Commission (NRC) regulates the commercial and institutional uses of nuclear material, including its use in diagnostic and clinical imaging. Established in 1974 following the abolition of the Atomic Energy Commission, the NRC now has six program offices, including the Office of Federal and State Materials and Environmental Management Program that oversees academic and medical uses.

The NRC's primary activities center on (a) establishing standards, regulations, and requirements related to the possession, use, and disposal of nuclear materials; (b) licensing facilities that are involved in these activities; and (c) inspecting these facilities to ensure compliance. In 36 states and one city (as of 2009), the NRC has relinquished responsibility for implementation to the state governments, referred to as Agreement States. The Agreement States issue radioactive material licenses, establish laws compatible with NRC regulations, and enforce those laws under the states' authority. For example, the Ohio Radiation Protection Programs covers both nuclear materials safety—including licensing, inspection, responding to radiologic incidents—and tracking low-level radioactive waste; and X-ray safety, which registers and inspects facilities with X-ray devices and linear accelerators and enforces the MQSA. Inspections of radiation generating equipment by health physicists include performance of compliance tests of exposure and timer reproducibility, half-value layer determination, and evaluation of human radiation safety. In non-Agreement States, the NRC is responsible for monitoring the use of nuclear material, while the Occupational Safety and Health Administration (OSHA) oversees all other ionizing radiation sources, including X-ray devices and linear accelerators.

Every time a radiation producing device is installed, moved, or upgraded, the appropriate registration agency must be updated, a key activity when seeking to set or revise the scope of service. The failure to meet NRC/state standards, including timely registration, may lead to fines and loss of the license for the radioactive materials.

Occupational Safety and Health Administration

The Occupational Safety and Health Administration (OSHA) has a broad mandate to prevent work-related injuries, illnesses, and deaths. Created in 1971 within the US Department of Labor, the agency provides free onsite assistance to identify and correct workplace hazards as well as training in job safety and health for employees through state and regional offices. It also carries out onsite inspections of workplaces, based on incidents of multiple worker deaths or injuries, employee complaints, reports from other agencies, or employer reports of significant levels of worker illness or injury. Since its creation, occupational deaths in the United States have been reduced by 62% and injuries by 42%.[7]

As is the case with the NRC, states can establish their own worker safety programs, which if approved by OSHA, assume responsibility for enforcing the OSHA standards. More than half of states and two US territories have OSHA approved programs. In 2006, OSHA and the state programs carried out over 96,000 inspections.[7]

OSHA regulations for general employee health and safety must be met. Repetitive stress injuries are the largest single category of injury in the workplace.[8] Among imaging professionals, sonographers have the highest rate of repetitive injury, with 84% experiencing work-related pain at some point in their careers.[9] Among the tasks that put imaging workers at greatest risk of injury are patient transfer and positioning, cassette handling, computer ergonomics, and equipment transfer.[10]

In addition to advising on and monitoring general worker health and safety, OSHA has special responsibilities relevant to the imaging facility. As noted above, while the NRC oversees activities related to nuclear materials, OSHA oversees the safe use of other ionizing radiation materials and devices. To keep all employees' exposure to radiation as low as reasonably achievable (known as ALARA), OSHA recommends a range of solutions including:

- The use of personnel monitoring devices (eg, film badges)
- A barrier wall with lead plated glass, behind which an employee can stand while operating an X-ray device
- Lead aprons for patients and/or employees within the direct X-ray field
- Proper maintenance of devices, with one or more employees specifically responsible
- Maintenance of radiation exposure records for all employees wearing personnel monitoring devices

OSHA is a valuable partner and resource. However, employers who violate the agency's regulations are subject to a range of penalties: (a) a citation with a time frame within which the violation must be corrected; (b) financial penalties, which can be substantial, with willful and repeat violations subject to penalties up to $70,000; and (c) liability for civil and/or criminal prosecution for violations that lead to serious health consequences or death of one or more workers.

State and Local Regulations

As has been noted, many states have programs that regulate worker health and safety and the nuclear medicine industry in lieu of the relevant federal programs. In such instances, the state programs must conform at least to the federal standards and, consequently, so must the facilities they monitor.

Among the other areas commonly regulated by states are the qualifications of professional and technical staff. According to the Bureau of Labor Statistics, 32 states license radiation therapists, 40 states require radiographers to be licensed, and more than half of all states license sonographers.[11] In Ohio, for example, radiographers, nuclear medicine technologists, radiation therapists, and general X-ray machine operators must successfully pass a state licensing examination. In some instances, states also require certification by the American Registry of Radiologic Technologists (ARRT).

State and local agencies, including health, building, and tax departments, may have other regulations that impact decisions about an imaging facility's scope of service. If service changes or additions entail renovations, for example, building codes that apply to both general construction and radiologic specific facilities must be identified and met. Health departments may have regulations about blood-borne pathogens and infection control that can affect the way in which a service is provided.

Develop Appropriate Services

Devising a list of potential services and identifying the regulatory issues that will have to be resolved to ensure compliance are important precursors to establishing a facility's scope of service. Consultation with the radiologists and staff members will help to further refine the process. In particular, developing appropriate services calls for an understanding of the clinical applications of modalities currently installed and proposed; efficient and effective management of all resources; and creation of technique charts and detailed policies and procedures.

Understand Clinical Applications of Modalities

If an imaging facility is to consistently provide services that patients need and insurers will pay for, the capabilities and limitations of current modalities must be understood, as well as their probable future uses and those of developing technologies. For example, mammography helped reduce the mortality rate from breast cancer by 20% during the final decade of the twentieth century, largely because of its usefulness as a screening tool to detect early cancer.[12] Yet its limitations include a 20% false-negative rate, inadequate detection in women with dense breast tissue, and an inability to distinguish between benign and cancerous breast lesions.[12]

As a result, a number of alternatives are in various stages of development and implementation, including contrast enhanced mammography and full field digital mammography (FFDM). In addition, developments in molecular biology are leading researchers in a new direction, producing images that measure regional tumor biology via noninvasive molecular assays. Each has its advantages and disadvantages and some may be less useful as screening tools than as diagnostic devices (Table 1.1). Nevertheless, one or more of these developments can be expected to become standard and working with the staff radiologists to assess when and how services utilizing them should be added to the facility's services.

Table 1.1 Advantages and Disadvantages of Modalities Used in Molecular Breast Imaging

Modality	*Advantages*	*Disadvantages*
Magnetic resonance (MR)		
MR imaging	High spatial resolution and image detail Increasing range of contrast agents under development	Confined space Contrast design limited by need for magnetic atom
MR spectroscopy	Can measure wide range of molecules No contrast needed	Limited spatial resolution Challenging to get high quality spectra in routine imaging
Radiocuclide imaging		
Positron emission tomography (PET)	Wide range of molecular imaging probes Tracer imaging without perturbing biological system	Limited spatial resolution Some radiation exposure
Single photon emission tomography	Similar to PET Probes more widely available	Less quantitatively accurate than PET
Ultrasound, especially with contrast enhancement	Highly portable, inexpensive Molecular microbubble contrast agents possible	Operator dependence Contrast agents confined to vascular space thus far
Optical imaging	Highly portable, inexpensive High spatial resolution possible	Limited penetration from surface; limited to relatively superficial sites

Source: Mankoff DA. Molecular imaging as a tool for translating breast cancer science. *Breast Cancer Res*. 2008;10(Suppl 1):S3-14. Available at: http://breast-cancer-research.com/content/10/S1/S3. Accessed July 21, 2009.

The limitations of ultrasound in the face of a changing patient population provide another example of the need to fully understand and appreciate the applications of a modality now and in the near future. With more than a third of the US adult population categorized as obese,[13] the inability of ultrasound to produce high quality images of fatty tissues has meant that facilities with traditional ultrasound devices are unable to effectively examine an increasing number of patients. Technological developments are offering two solutions. The first, differential tissue harmonics imaging, allows the simultaneous transmission of two frequencies within the same pulse, providing superior border and tissue definition. The second is 4-D imaging, which takes multiple ultrasound images in rapid succession and produces a 3-D motion video.[14]

Here are some suggestions of ways to ensure maximum clinical usefulness of all modalities, now and in the near future:

1. In consultation with lead technologists in each modality, a spreadsheet can be created for each modality, listing the tests currently being performed, their function as diagnostic or therapeutic, the types of patients using them, the rate of incomplete tests or poor quality images, and the reasons for problems. Updated on a quarterly or semiannual basis, these charts may reveal trends that could be used to target modality changes (eg, an increase in the number of patients with diabetes over 65 years old undergoing ultrasound of their feet for detection of decreased arterial blood flow). Use of advanced Doppler technology in these patients can decrease the rate of lower extremity amputation.[14]
2. Technologists for each modality should be encouraged to review the respective literature on an ongoing basis and draw attention to new developments.
3. Staff members who attend professional conferences should be charged with monitoring discussions of new services and technological developments and producing a summary for planning purposes.
4. Reservations staff can be trained to report requests for tests not currently performed at the facility as a starting point to analyze the tests' potential addition to the scope of service.
5. A focus group or survey of referring physicians (or of physicians who should be referring but are not) can probe for unmet needs.

Manage Resources to Achieve Service Plans

Maintaining an effective scope of service requires a balance among the necessary resources—staff, finances, equipment, and supplies. A head count that is top heavy with clerical staff but lacks sufficient sonographers will fail to meet the patients' ultrasound needs. Equipment that is idle because relevant supplies are not on hand wastes financial and human resources. Gaps in cash flow may lead to layoffs or delayed maintenance with the potential to negatively affect service delivery.

A study of more than 400 hospital imaging departments found that many of these departments were operating far below their potential capacity.[15] Among the factors leading to this suboptimal performance were:

- Leaders who focused on capital investment rather than operations
- Understaffing and underscheduling
- Poorly aligned financial incentives
- A fragmented view of operations

These could be translated as failures to properly manage human resources, financial resources, and equipment and supplies. The other books in this AHRA series discuss these topics in depth.

Develop Technique Charts

Safe radiological examinations involve factors that are subject to variation. These include factors related to the patient (eg, weight, disease state), the operator (eg, experience, training), and the equipment (eg, default settings, radiation levels). Successfully delivering services that meet customer needs calls for achieving consistency in image quality. Among the ways to accomplish this are to develop policies and procedures that every employee must follow with every patient and to create technique charts that take into account equipment and patient variability.

Technique charts take into consideration the role of the primary factors of peak kilovolts (kV[p]), milliamperes (mA), exposure time (S), and/or mAS, as well as secondary factors of distance from the source of radiation to the film (source to image distance [SID]), the types of grids being used, and whether the system is film based or digital. The penetrating ability of the X-rays is dependent on the level of kVp; the optimum level produces images with enough contrast to provide the radiologist with the most information. The patient's total radiation exposure is controlled by mA, S (or mAS), and SID; the goal is to use settings that produce the best image with the lowest radiation exposure. Both S and mAS need to be adjusted for patient size.

Because the actual radiation coming from the X-ray source varies among devices, a set of technique charts must be created for each radiography room, mobile device, or exam protocol. Typically, a basic set would include charts for:

- Adult chest
- Adult extremities
- Adult shoulder/knee
- Adult ribs
- Adult lumbar spine/pelvis/hip/femur
- Adult thoracic spine
- Adult cervical spine
- Infant chest
- Child spine
- Child skull/sinus/facial bones
- Pediatric extremity

Figures 1.1 and 1.2 show examples of chest, extremity, and shoulder/knee technique charts for a film-based system and a digital one, respectively.

Templates for technique charts may be available from the equipment manufacturer or other resources. These templates can be customized using phantoms supplied by the equipment manufacturer or water phantoms created with plastic shoeboxes and water. An amount of 6 cm (2.3 inches) of water in a single box can represent a forearm; 15 cm (5.8 inches) is equivalent to the lumbar spine. The technologist follows the standard procedure for placement of film cassette and exposure of film.

To assess the result in a film-based system, the technologist places a newspaper under the processed film; using ordinary room light, if the newsprint is barely visible through the image of the water, the density (and thus the settings) is appropriate. If the newsprint can be clearly seen through the image, S or mAS needs to be increased; if the newsprint cannot be seen, then S or mAS needs to be decreased. For a digital system, the resulting image will be displayed on the workstation monitor with an exposure data recognition number. This number should fall within the manufacturer's guidelines supplied with the equipment. If not, the S or mAS should be adjusted according to the device manual.

For either system, tests should be repeated until the appropriate density is achieved, at which point the settings can be recorded in the technique chart. The proportion

Typical Film/Screen Imaging Chart

Manual Timed Exposures Guideline
Medium-High Frequency equipment
12:1 table Bucky; 10:1 vertical Bucky
400/100 film/screen imaging

RADIOGRAPHIC OPERATIONS CONSULTING

Typical output
60 kVp 2.5-3.0 mR/mAS
80 kVp 5.0-6.0 mR/mAS
110 kVp 10-12 mR/mAS

CHEST PA & Lat 8:1 - 10:1 Grid - *typical high frequency/400 speed imaging*

CM 72" SID	16	20	24	28	32	36	40
kVp	90	110	110	110	110	110	110
mAS	1.5	1.5	3.0	6.0	12	24	48
NON GRID	76 kVp 0.75 mAS	80 kVp Same mAS					

EXTREMITIES *typical high-frequency 100 speed/400 speed - tabletop*

CM typical anatomy 40" SID	1-2 digits	3-4 PA hand, PA wrist, distal foot	5-7 Lat wrist, forearm, prox foot, lat ankle	8-9 elbow, AP ankle, lower leg	10-11 humerus, knee
kVp	56	60	60	60	60
▶ mAS 100 speed	1.5	2.0	3.0	4.0-5.0	6.0
▶ mAS 400 speed	52 kVp 1.0 mAS	56 kVp 1.0 mAS	60 kV @ 1.0	60 kV @ 1.5	60 kV @ 2.0

SHOULDER/KNEE *typical high-frequency 400 speed - 10/12:1 Bucky/grid*

CM 40" SID	9-10	11-12	13-14	15-16	
kVp	80	80	80	80	
mAS	1.5	2.0	3.0	4.0	
Axial shoulder	Clavicle with 25° tilt	Trans thoracic	Scapular Y view	Tangential knee	Tunnel knee
no grid 70-72 kVp 1.0 mAS	multiply AP mAS by 1.5	measure chest and humerus 80 kVp 36 cm 80mAS 40 cm 160mAS	80 kVp 6-8 mAS	no grid 80 kVp 60" SID 5 mAS 40" SID 2.5	with Bucky about same as AP no grid multiply AP mAS by 0.2

Figure 1.1 Three Examples of Technique Charts for a Typical Film-Based X-Ray System

Source: Radiographic Room Handbook. Aurora, NE: Radiographic Operations Consulting; 2008: 25. Used with permission.

Typical Digital Imaging Chart 1

Manual Timed Exposures Guideline
Medium-High Frequency equipment
12:1 table Bucky; 10:1 vertical Bucky
Digital Imaging—nominal 100" speed for extremeties and 400 for all else

RADIOGRAPHIC OPERATIONS CONSULTING

Typical output
60 kVp 2.5-3.0 mR/mAS
80 kVp 5.0-6.0 mR/mAS
110 kVp 10-12 mR/mAS

CHEST PA & Lat—*8:1—10:1 grid*

CM 72" SID	15	20	25	30	35	40	45
kVp	120	120	120	120	120	120	120
mAS	1.2	2.5	5.0	10	20	40	80
NON GRID	86 kVp Same mAS						

EXTREMITIES—*100 "speed" tabletop*

CM typical anatomy 40" SID	1-2 digits	3-4 PA hand, PA wrist, distal foot	5-7 Lat wrist, forearm, prox foot, lat ankle	8-9 elbow, AP ankle, lower leg	10-11 humerus, knee
kVp	60	60	60	60	60
mAS	1.0	2.0	3.0	4.0-5.0	6.0

SHOULDER/KNEE—*Table or Wall Bucky/grid*

CM 40" SID	9-10	11-12	13-14	15-16	
kVp	80	80	80	80	
mAS	3.0	4.0	6.0	8.0	
Axial shoulder	Clavicle with 25° tilt	Trans thoracic	Scapular Y view	Tangential knee	Tunnel knee
no grid 70-72 kVp 2.0 mAS	multiply AP mAS by 1.5	measure chest and humerus 80 kVp 36 cm 100 mAS 40 cm 200 mAS	80 kVp 10-12 mAS	no grid 80 kVp 60" SID 8.0 mAS 40" SID 4.0	with Bucky about same as AP no grid multiply AP mAS by 0.2

Figure 1.2 Three Examples of Technique Charts for a Typical Digital X-Ray System

Source: Radiographic Room Handbook. Aurora, NE: Radiographic Operations Consulting; 2008: 30. Used with permission.

of change in S or mAS for the phantom test should be applied to all the values within a given chart, that is, if the best extremity image was produced with an mAS that is double that of the template for 6 cm, then all mAS values for the extremity should be doubled.[16]

The preparation of technique charts is best done when the device is newly calibrated and the film processor is clean (for film-based systems). The charts should be reassessed whenever the equipment undergoes major repair work or is moved. Copies of the charts should be kept with the relevant device in the radiography room and in the policies and procedures manual. The technologist should record the settings used in the patient's file.

Conclusion

Nothing in healthcare is static. Certainly, this is true for the services an imaging facility supplies to its patients and their referring physicians. Preparations must be made to reassess the facility's scope of service frequently, based on changes in customer needs, government regulations, reimbursement policies, and imaging technology.

References

1. US Department of Health & Human Services. Summary of the HIPAA Privacy Rule. http://www.hhs.gov/ocr/privacy/hipaa/understanding/summary/index.html. Revised May 3, 2009. Accessed July 1, 2009.

2. US Department of Health & Human Services. Health information privacy complaints received by calendar year. http://www.hhs.gov/ocr/privacy/hipaa/enforcement/data/complaintsyear.html. Accessed July 17, 2009.

3. Centers for Medicare & Medicaid Services. Security 101 for covered entities. HIPAA Security Series, Vol. 2, Paper 1. Revised March 2007. Available at: http://www.hhs.gov/ocr/privacy/hipaa/administrative/securityrule/security101.pdf. Accessed March 17, 2010.

4. Food and Drug Administration. Mammography facility adverse event and action report—2008. http://www.fda.gov/downloads/Radiation-EmittingProducts/MammographyQualityStandardsActandProgram/Reports/ucm124183.pdf. Published March 6, 2009. Accessed July 16, 2009.

5. *Ambulatory Care Accreditation Handbook*. Oak Terrace, IL: Joint Commission on Accreditation of Healthcare Organizations; 2009:5–6.

6. National Committee for Quality Assurance. About NCQA. http://www.ncqa.org/tabid/675/Default.aspx. Accessed July 1, 2009.

7. Occupational Safety & Health Administration. Frequently asked questions. http://www.osha.gov/html/comp-links-faq.html. Accessed March 17, 2010.

8. Webster T. Putting a strain on worker's health. *Compensation and Working Conditions*, Bureau of Labor Statistics. Spring 1999. http://www.bls.gov/opub/cwc/archive/spring1999brief2.pdf. Accessed August 4, 2009.

9. Pike I, Russo A, Berkowitz J, Baker J, Lessoway V. The prevalence of musculoskeletal disorders among diagnostic medical sonographers. *JDMS*. 1997; 13:219–227.

10. Murphey SL. Reducing work related injuries through participatory work safety programs. *Radiol Manage*. 2009;31(1):35–41.

11. Radiation therapists. In: *Occupational Outlook Handbook 2008–09*. Washington, DC: Bureau of Labor Statistics; 2008. Available at: www.bls.gov/oco/ocos299.htm. Accessed June 25, 2009.

12. Smith AP, Hall PA, Marcello DM. Emerging technologies in breast cancer detection. *Radiol Manage*. 2004;26(4):16–24.

13. Ogden CL, Carroll MD, McDowell MA, Flegal KM. Obesity among adults in the United States—no statistically significant change since 2003–2004. Centers for Disease Control and Prevention, National Ceneters for Health Statistics Data Sheet. http://www.cdc.gov/nchs/data/databriefs/db01.pdf. Revised December 2007. Accessed August 4, 2009.

14. Parhar G. Advances in ultrasound move modality into new fields. *Radiol Manage*. 2006;28(2):34–41.

15. Joffe S, Drew D, Bansal M, Hase M. Radiology operations: what you don't know could be costing you millions. *Radiol Manage*. 2007;29(4):20–24.

16. *Radiographic Room Handbook*. Aurora, NE: Radiographic Operations Consulting; 2008. Available at: www.controlthedose.com.

Chapter 2

Build Alliances

Suzanne K. Ramthun, Sue A. Rysted, and Kathleen J. Williams

The ability of imaging facilities to align themselves with others is an essential component of a successful operation. Alliances can take various forms, including internal organizational imaging practice service lines (eg, cardiology, gastroenterology), industry partnerships (eg, pharmaceutical research), referring provider alliances, and joint ventures. This chapter provides guidelines for identifying alliance opportunities and appropriate partners; highlights issues particularly relevant to forming and maintaining effective alliances; discusses legal issues; and describes techniques to ensure ongoing communication among partners.

Strategic alliances and collaborative partnerships allow businesses to work jointly to achieve mutually beneficial objectives and leverage their strengths for effectiveness.[1] Organizations form strategic alliances and partnerships to support their planned initiatives, strengthen their resources, and remain competitive in the industry.[2] Large or small, healthcare organizations have concluded that to remain competitive requires a diverse and knowledgeable workforce, access to technology and technological expertise, and efficient business practices. Business alliances can be an effective way to combine the best features of the partners, enabling them to achieve more than if they functioned entirely alone.

As used in this chapter, alliances are formal agreements between two or more business entities (eg, departments, practices, pharmaceutical companies, imaging centers) to pursue specific goals while remaining independent. In particular, these alliances usually accomplish one or more of the following[1]:

1. They are critical to achieving an organization's strategic objectives.
2. They help build, sustain, or enhance competitive advantage.
3. They block a competitive threat.
4. They open new opportunities to expand services or markets.
5. They mitigate a significant risk to the business.

Whether as a hospital-based imaging department or a freestanding imaging center, providing diagnostic or clinical imaging services involves myriad internal and external relationships (Figure 2.1). As shown in the Venn diagram, the patient is central to imaging operations. Imaging employees, patient clinical services, and referring

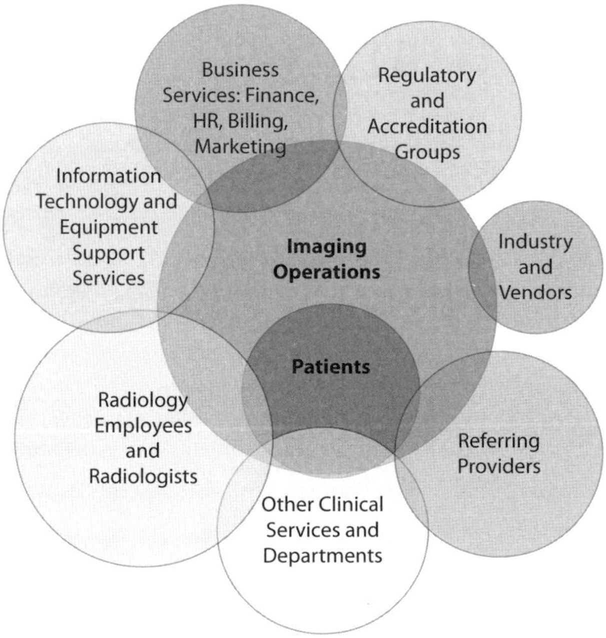

Figure 2.1 Venn Diagram Illustrating Typical Radiology Operations Interrelationships

providers work directly to provide patient services and care, while information technology, business services, regulatory groups, and industry vendors influence imaging operations and patient care.

The patient is also central to many alliances, which may be formed between one or more of the groups with existing relationships. A medical oncology group, for example, may ally with a radiation oncology group to provide both diagnostic and therapeutic services. The same radiologists perform all examinations, so reporting is consistent and meets the oncologists' needs. Patients may experience better coordination of their care and easier access to healthcare services when diagnostic and clinical services are centralized.[3]

Other alliances may be formed with an industry partner (eg, pharmaceutical company), for example, to carry out joint research to develop a new imaging technology or design new imaging protocols. Still another form of strategic alliance may involve collaboration between imaging and other departments within an institution. In both cases, a good working relationship between the departments or organizations is essential for business success. When forming a strategic alliance, each organization should expect to share resources, risks, and rewards resulting from the alliance.

A strategic alliance may be a wise approach when organizations are faced with fast paced, high priced technological developments, enabling partners to develop ancillary services they could not have developed on their own. Additionally, strategic alliances help lower costs through shared resources including personnel, expertise, and training programs. For example, an imaging group and a hospital may form a joint venture to purchase and operate an MRI scanner or PET device. Such an alliance achieves not only patient care goals, but financial goals as well by both lowering costs and adding a new revenue stream.

Alliances such as group purchasing arrangements are another way to achieve financial goals. Through group purchasing efforts, partners can negotiate from a position of strength, achieving lower costs and, in some cases, better products and/or services.

Alliances such as trade or exchange agreements allow participating organizations to focus their resources on providing their products or services at highly efficient levels.[4] An organization can gain a comparative advantage when it can focus its resources on its core competencies and efficiently produce products or services at a lower cost or a lower opportunity cost than other organizations. On the other hand, an organization is at a comparative disadvantage if higher real costs or opportunity costs result from providing certain products or services. Therefore, it is a wise business strategy to form alliances for the exchange of products or services in areas for which both comparative advantages and disadvantages exist. Overall, it pays to explore business alliances that can lead to new and innovative methods for providing quality services to customers efficiently and effectively.

Alliances such as those described above differ from straightforward business transactions in a number of ways. In particular, transactions (eg, licensing, outsourcing) tend to be based solely on a contract, which spells out all rights and responsibilities. This leaves little opportunity for creative problem solving within the relationship. Each party is focused on what it can get from the transaction, rather than on achieving mutual goals, and neither party has regard for the well-being of the other. Information sharing tends to be minimal—only what is needed to complete the transaction. Outcomes tend to be one time events or short-term arrangements.

On the other hand, while contracts or other formal agreements are necessary in alliances, the dynamic nature of the relationship means that not every detail can be spelled out in advance. Successful alliances may make use of transactions as part of their tactics, but usually go far beyond to function as true partnerships that[1,5]:

- Are based on an understanding that neither partner benefits by hurting the other
- Involve mutual sharing of information (within predetermined parameters) and other key resources

- Are respectful of the culture and business practices of each partner
- Are flexible enough to allow creative problem solving and adaptations to achieve ongoing improvements beyond what could be achieved with a transaction
- Are structured so that decisions can be made swiftly, especially in response to technological advancements or changes in the healthcare environment
- Agree that the objective is important and that it can best be achieved by the alliance
- Acknowledge that each partner brings significant value to the other and to the alliance project
- Allow each partner to concentrate on its core competencies while learning other competencies from each other that may be used elsewhere

Evaluate Alliance Options

Once an organization has identified its key objectives, it can begin evaluating the various types of alliances to determine which, if any, will best achieve those objectives. The three general types are direct cooperation, joint ventures, and minority investments.

Direct Cooperation

Direct cooperation, also referred to as a nonequity strategic alliance, requires two or more entities to share some of their unique resources and/or capabilities to achieve mutual objectives. Operating links are formed without substantial integration into each partner's other operations. Direct cooperation is the simplest alliance to form, which makes it the most common. Its simplicity also means it can usually be formed in less time and can more easily be dissolved than the other two types.

On the other hand, these qualities make direct cooperation unsuitable to achieve certain objectives, such as the goal of creating a separate organization that will require financial investment in infrastructure. Projects that call for substantial integration of both partners' activities are also not candidates for direct cooperation, nor are those that involve a significant departure from the partners' core competencies.

Examples of direct cooperation within healthcare include:

- Group purchasing organizations
- Collaboration between a hospital-based imaging department and an imaging device manufacturer to develop new protocols or product improvements
- Participation in clinical trials to determine diagnostic or treatment efficacy
- Joint marketing effort by two hospital departments

Joint Ventures

Two or more partners form a joint venture when they want to create a separate legal entity to achieve their objective(s). The new business has its own staff, with senior staff pulled from the partner businesses. This staffing model is to ensure the venture has the intellectual capital it needs and management understands the partners' objectives. Resources may be purchased by the new business or be provided by the partners. Of course, the new business offers a product or service that separately the partners cannot or do not wish to provide, and its markets may be different from those of the partners.

Joint ventures can be structured in one of three ways.

> The first joint venture structure has full equality participation. Each organization usually has 50%–50% ownership and the partners share equally in all policy and operating issues. This form is generally used when (a) both partners have critical expertise to contribute on an ongoing basis; (b) ongoing coordination is essential; or (c) the partners are rivals who have decided to collaborate for this particular project alone.
>
> The second joint venture structure is one of policy equality. In such cases, both partners share equally in all policy decisions and ownership, but one partner handles day-to-day operations of the joint venture. This structure is best used when both partners have essential expertise, but the new business retains the expertise of one partner over the other.
>
> Finally, the third joint venture structure is the lead partner venture, in which one partner is responsible for most policy matters and all operational activities of the new business. The minority partner has veto over specified issues. The ownership proportions can vary, but usually the lead partner has a majority financial stake in the project. Lead partner ventures are most applicable in situations in which (a) the partners have divergent management styles that make close cooperation difficult; (b) one partner does not need to contribute expertise on an ongoing basis; or (c) the minority partner's interest is operational, not strategic.[5]

Full equality ventures require that the partners reach consensus on all key policy and operational issues, which can make managing the business difficult. At the same time, when both partners have an equal say, they are more likely to make their best effort on behalf of the project. Nevertheless, unless circumstances warrant, the lead partner structure is preferable.[5]

Examples of joint ventures in healthcare include:

- A medical oncology group, an imaging group, a surgical practice, and a women's spa create a women's breast cancer center
- An imaging center and a medical device manufacturer form a venture to commercialize a device developed by the center's lead radiologist
- A hospital and a freestanding imaging center create a PET center

Minority Investment

The least common form of alliance is one that involves one partner investing in another, usually smaller, partner. The investor owns less than 50% of the other business and does not have operational or policy control, although in return for the financing, the investor may have one or more seats on the governing board. Such an alliance provides much needed capital to the smaller business, which may also benefit from the investor's management expertise or industry contacts. The investor business gets access to the smaller business's key expertise or resources, ideally to meet its objective(s) at lower costs or with fewer operational issues than if the investor chose to develop the expertise or resources on their own. Although the investor's ultimate expectation is to gain financially, the primary focus is on achieving a strategic advantage.

To succeed, a minority investment should be made in a business that is strong and well managed. Its business scope should be narrow and focused on objectives that are to the mutual benefit of both partners. Although the investor has no direct control over policy or operations, it expects a cooperative relationship that acknowledges its right to be heard. These investments will usually involve alliances designed to operate for several years.

Healthcare minority investments might include:

- A device manufacturer that provides funds to a radiologist to complete initial testing on a new device he or she has invented
- An imaging center that invests in a small diagnostic laboratory that will provide onsite testing services to the center's patients
- A rural hospital that invests in the first imaging practice to offer MRI services in its community

Some Techniques to Evaluate Alliance Options

In seeking to achieve various strategic and business objectives, an imaging facility has a wide range of options—straightforward transactions, the three alliance types, or even mergers and acquisitions. The best alternative must be determined before seeking out an alliance partner.

One tool in the evaluation process is the cost-benefit analysis, which monetizes the potential benefits and costs related to a project and calculates the net result (Table 2.1).[6] Even when the primary objective of a potential alliance is not financial, performing a cost-benefit analysis can be useful to establish at least a break-even point. For purposes of evaluating alliance options or other major projects, the cost-benefit analysis focuses on future cash expenditures and relevant benefits that result from the decision to proceed.[7] In other words, the costs to be considered are:

- Cash outlays (do not include opportunity or other intangible costs)
- Future costs, generally from the start of project implementation (do not include costs of items being repurposed for the project)
- Direct results of the project (do not include fixed expenses that would be made with or without the project)

Usually, the costs can be more accurately calculated than the benefits, as the costs are often an extension or duplication of current costs. The benefits to be considered must be directly associated with the project and, in most cases, will be a projection of increased revenues. If the market is in flux, it may be useful to perform the analysis using several revenue scenarios (eg, if revenues increased by 5%, 15%, or 50%).

In addition to conducting a cost-benefit analysis of the most promising options, other issues should be compared such as[5]:

- Level of investment that will be required and probable source(s)
- Resources needed and probable source(s)
- Potential risks involved
- Time required to make the project operational and whether this meets objectives
- Level of strategic or operational control sought
- Level of integration into existing organization sought

An important consideration before selecting an option is healthcare market trends. An alliance that seeks to increase patient volume and/or revenues, for example, relies on the assumption that demand will continue as expected and that past performance is a good indicator of future performance. This is

Table 2.1 Cost-Benefit Analysis for Hypothetical Joint Purchase of Capital Equipment

	Year 1	*Year 2*	*Year 3*	*Year 4*	*Year 5*	*Total*
Benefits						
Additional revenue	$3,600,000	$4,000,000	$4,400,000	$4,900,000	$5,400,000	$ 22,300,000
Costs						
Equipment (cash purchase)	–$1,500,000	0	0	0	0	–$ 1,500,000
Service Contract	0	–$ 100,000	–$ 100,000	–$ 100,000	–$ 100,000	–$ 400,000
Renovations	–$ 125,000	0	0	0	0	–$ 125,000
Operating costs (administrative, etc)	–$ 30,000	–$ 31,000	–$ 32,000	–$ 34,000	–$ 35,000	–$ 162,000
Cost of sales (salaries, supplies, etc)	–$ 249,000	–$ 260,000	–$ 350,000	–$ 361,000	–$ 378,000	–$ 1,598,000
Discounts (bad debts, etc) @ 55%	–$1,980,000	–$2,200,000	–$2,420,000	–$2,700,000	–$2,970,000	–$ 12,270,000
Net cash flow	–$ 284,000	$1,409,000	$1,498,000	$1,705,000	$1,917,000	$ 6,245,000

relatively accurate only if few or no changes in key parameters (eg, service quality) are made. An alliance that affects the cost or perceived quality of the service or product may affect the predictability of future business. Furthermore, external changes—such as in healthcare regulations, insurance coverage, competing imaging facilities, or the overall economy—may result in variations in the demand for services. A decline in the overall economy, for example, may have little impact on demand for services for emergency and life threatening conditions, but screenings and other more elective services may experience a decline as patients forgo seeking treatment. These trends are not always easy to predict, often making estimating future performance a best guess, but an estimate worth making nonetheless.

Identify Potential Alliance Partners

Once the decision has been made that an alliance is the best way to achieve the planned objectives, one or more partners must be approached for their willingness to ally. In addition to meeting the criteria for successful alliances outlined earlier, partner organizations should have the following characteristics[5]:

- Collaborative ethos—Organizations that have a proven record of encouraging collaboration among their employees have the necessary skills to collaborate externally.
- Management by objectives—Organizations that manage by objectives are better able to incorporate alliance objectives into their internal operations.
- Compatible culture—Partners need to have business cultures that suit the alliance and are compatible with each other. A heavily bureaucratic organization, for example, will not be a suitable partner in an alliance that requires speed and flexibility.
- Relationship builders—A hallmark of alliances is the reliance on personal relationships, particularly among the senior management, that encourage full disclosure, honesty, frankness, and a willingness to reach consensus on key issues. More problems in alliances are due to weak relationships than to anything else.
- Change agents—Alliance leaders from each of the partner groups need a proven record of successfully leading change, as nearly all alliances will ultimately produce ongoing advances that translate into operational changes.
- Team builders—Alliance policy leaders need to establish a shared vision for the project; give clear and consistent guidance to operational staff; be willing to share detailed information, responsibilities, risks, and rewards; and meld a functioning team from both organizations.

A search should begin within a current network, where recognizing the above characteristics is easier than with total strangers. Among the possible sources are current suppliers, including device manufacturers, laboratories, and pharmaceutical firms; other healthcare providers who may be referring patients or with whom the radiologists serve on hospital committees; and hospitals with which the radiologists are affiliated. Local universities, especially those with medical schools or programs to train nurses and other allied health professionals, may be suitable partners. A hospital-based imaging department can also look to other departments within the facility or to its affiliated organizations (eg, a for-profit equipment service business or a rehabilitation center within the umbrella of a hospital holding company).

Clarify Issues for Effective Working Relationships

Once a potential alliance partner has been identified, preliminary discussions should begin to flesh out the myriad details that will help ensure objectives are achieved (Sidebar 2.1). Among the early issues that should be raised are:

SIDEBAR 2.1: A Checklist for Alliance Negotiations

- ✓ Confirm that identified leaders can deliver in the name of their organization and will be held accountable for the alliance.
- ✓ Agree on alliance ethics.
- ✓ Define a shared alliance vision based on each partner's objective(s).
- ✓ Agree on financial sharing principles.
- ✓ Identify and assign team members for daily activities.
- ✓ Build a shared understanding of each partner's strengths, practices, skills, and legal contexts.
- ✓ Define conflict resolution procedures.
- ✓ Determine adequate safeguards for information sharing.
- ✓ Begin managing expectations about outcomes between partners and beyond the alliance.
- ✓ Identify alliance activities, checking for completeness in obtaining mutual objectives.
- ✓ Determine negotiation timetable.
- ✓ Perform joint marketing and technical research to establish opportunities.
- ✓ Develop a joint business plan.
- ✓ Agree on suppliers.
- ✓ Outline separate and joint financial models for alliance.
- ✓ Agree on specifics for sharing costs, benefits, and risks.
- ✓ Involve legal representation for each partner.
- ✓ Align within each partner organization.
- ✓ Create a governing body.
- ✓ Plan for termination agreement.

Source: Adapted from Lewis JD. *Trusted Partners: How Companies Build Mutual Trust and Win Together.* New York, NY: The Free Press; 1999.

- What objective(s) does each partner believe the alliance can achieve, including so called stretch objectives that reflect "above and beyond" accomplishments?
- What resources is each partner prepared to contribute?
- What issues must be resolved before the alliance can be implemented?
- What issues, if any, are deal breakers for either partner?
- If an opportunity arises, can partners discuss alliance options with other potential partners, and at what point would such discussions no longer be allowed?
- Who will the policy and operational leaders be for the alliance from each partner?
- What are the potential net benefits?

These preliminary discussions are also the time to begin building the open relationships that will be critical to the success of the alliance. As soon as the joint leaders are identified, they should begin taking part in not only formal discussions but also informal ones designed to build trust and increase knowledge of each other's way of thinking, making decisions, and managing.

Before discussions proceed beyond the preliminary phase, any legal or regulatory issues should be identified through consultation with attorneys. "The Stark law governing referrals, non-compete and antitrust regulations, licensing, and even health plan credentialing all have potential to penalize groups that fail to carry out due diligence."[3] See Sidebar 2.2.

The team will also want to develop a business plan for the alliance. Good business plans begin with the objectives and describe important resources, functions, products, services, finances, and sequencing of timing expectations. The plan should also include what will be expected from each partner through the collaboration. Some functions may be solely delegated to one partner, while others may be jointly carried out. The business plan should outline the scope, goals, and objectives and attempt to forecast the industry needs and trends over the life of the partnership. The business plan can be referenced as a reminder of the objective of the venture as needed. (For more details on creating business plans, see AHRA's book *Financial Management in Radiology*.)

Since alliances involve two or more partners in a shared enterprise (and each maintains their separate businesses), some unique issues related to trust, sharing, and management may arise.

Building Alliances on Trust

The partners need to rely on each other's character, integrity, and commitment if an alliance is to succeed. This is the very definition of trust, and both partners must be

SIDEBAR 2.2: Compliance with the Stark Law

A wide range of federal, state, and local regulations can affect whether an alliance can be formed and if so, how it can be structured. Especially for projects involving joint ownership and/or provision of services by healthcare organizations, one of the most relevant laws is Section 1877 of the Social Security Act, commonly referred to as the Stark Law.

The Stark Law, which has been implemented and amended in several phases, is an effort to tighten oversight of certain diagnostic imaging practices. In general, the law prohibits a physician from referring Medicare patients for designated services to entities with whom the physician (or the physicians immediate family members) has a financial relationship. There are a number of exceptions, including referrals by physicians who provide services to a primarily rural population, certain referrals by diagnostic radiologists, and referrals for invasive radiology procedures. In 2009, a series of changes were made, among which were:

- Prohibition of the use of compensation formulas for space and equipment leases that are based on percentage of revenue raised, billed, or otherwise related to the services performed.
- Expansion of the applicability of Stark to organizations that either bill Medicare for a service or provide that service; this will prohibit, for example, a referring physician from investing in a radiology practice that provides services to a hospital which then bills Medicare for those radiology services.

The Centers for Medicare and Medicaid Services, which interprets the Stark Law, reviews it on an ongoing basis, so legal advice is essential to ensure compliance with the latest amendments. For more about the Stark Law, visit http://starklaw.org.

willing to work at establishing and maintaining mutual trust from the very beginning of the relationship.

Below are eight conditions that nurture trust among partners[5]:

1. The mutual objective is a priority for each partner.
2. Strong interpersonal relationships enable conflict resolution and enhance performance.
3. Joint leaders collaborate and are role models.
4. Shared objectives guide alliance performance.
5. Safeguards (eg, policies regarding data sharing) encourage sharing and trust.
6. Commitment (eg, assigning the best people) and fairness create enthusiasm.
7. Adaptability enables the partners to work together.
8. Continuity of participants helps ensure alliance stability.

Among the techniques to build trust are to use logic, not politics, to guide problem solving; explore issues with an open mind before attempting to find a solution; be direct and candid; treat all participants as equals; and share benefits and risks fairly.

To Share or Not to Share

An alliance is unlikely to be effective if one partner believes it is shouldering more than its fair share of risk or is receiving less than its fair share of the benefits. Risks, costs, and benefits do not need to be shared equally (in fact, alliance structure will often dictate unequal shares), but they must be shared fairly. Early discussions are likely to center on assumptions that will guide cost allocations, pricing, and other key issues, as well as parameters that will be used to judge fairness. Depending on the alliance structure being considered, the negotiators can devise a sharing formula.

Before agreements are made, all parties should understand how assets will be valued and how benefits resulting from the alliance will be distinguished from benefits accruing to each partner's separate efforts. Benchmark data or third party valuations can be used to set values, if necessary. If the partners are investing jointly in an asset such as office space, principles guiding access should be outlined. Revenues will usually be shared based on the value of each partner's contribution to the alliance.

With regard to costs, the parties should agree on what will constitute alliance costs, how they will be shared, and what the charges will be. It may not be appropriate to reveal the partners' specific costs in some instances (eg, labor costs), in which case benchmark data or another nonproprietary source can be used to devise a full-time equivalent figure that both parties agree to use in calculating reimbursable costs.

Both parties should also agree on the information each organization will and will not share and develop policies that will govern proprietary data. For example, team members with access to sensitive data may be required to sign nondisclosure documents. Proprietary or sensitive data that is shared should be clearly marked "confidential" and access should be restricted to employees on a "need to know" basis. If computer access to data will be shared, each partner should have a security audit performed and any additional recommended measures in place before the alliance is implemented. Employees of each partner should be regularly reminded to restrict their data to alliance activities and refrain from sharing the information with anyone outside the alliance. Partners should also avoid sharing expertise methodology that relates to their core competence.

Respecting a partner's proprietary interests is just one of several ethical principles that should guide an alliance, as outlined in Sidebar 2.3.

SIDEBAR 2.3: Ethics for Alliances

All business transactions have rules that guide actions known as ethics, or a code of conduct. Some of these rules such as the need for honesty are widely embraced and generally applied. Others such as patient confidentiality may be specific to an industry or transaction. Below are six commonly accepted ethical rules that guide successful alliance activities:

1. **Identify deal breakers:** Early in discussions, negotiators should be upfront about any potential deal breakers—objectives or activities over which a partner is unwilling to compromise. As more information becomes available, some of these may cease to be deal breakers, but neither party should be blindsided by objections at the last minute.
2. **Honor previous obligations:** Obligations that were made before the alliance must be honored. Nothing should be part of an alliance that will cause either party to ignore commitments to others. Otherwise, the new partner's trust will erode.
3. **Disclose conflicts:** Starting with preliminary discussions, both parties should be honest and forthright about any conflicting objectives or other major issues that will need to be resolved. Partners should not deceive one another about elements fundamental to the alliance.
4. **Respect alliance boundaries:** Partners must respect each other's proprietary interests. Firewalls and other measures will provide some protection, but the close nature of many alliances means that sensitive information may be inadvertently revealed, which should never be shared with anyone or used in any way.
5. **Respect personnel boundaries:** Alliance partners should not recruit or hire employees from each other, if for no other reason than taking the firm's best staff members may negatively affect its performance and that of the alliance.
6. **Appraise of negative news:** A partner facing litigation, negative press, or other issues that could affect its image, finances, performance, or ability to meet alliance commitments should tell the other partner as soon as possible.

Source: Adapted from Lewis JD. *Trusted Partners: How Companies Build Mutual Trust and Win Together*. New York, NY: The Free Press; 1999.

Plan to Manage

The aphorism "the devil is in the details" is indeed true for discussions surrounding alliance governance and management. Even the simplest direct cooperation project requires the joint leaders and the planning team to reach consensus on myriad issues, not the least of which is how the alliance will be integrated with existing operations in both partner businesses. In the case of direct cooperation, employees carrying out alliance tasks will remain employees of the partners, but separate timekeeping will probably need to be implemented. For some joint venture projects, it may also be advisable to have a shared workspace to allow team interaction without interfering with the partners' separate businesses or revealing unrelated proprietary information. If a joint venture is being planned, key employees will come from the partners but in most cases should become employees of the venture without the ability to transfer back to the partner businesses. This encourages complete commitment to the joint venture.

Among the other management and governance issues to be considered before the alliance is implemented are:

1. **Decision making:** How will policy and operational decisions be made and by whom? How will disagreements be resolved? What will the approval process be for day-to-day operations?
2. **Oversight:** Is a separate governing board necessary? If so, who will sit on the board and what will its role be?
3. **Activities:** What will be the alliance activities? How do they relate to the mutual objectives? Which alliance activities will each partner carry out? What will be the alliance scope? What activities will the partners continue to carry out separate from the alliance? Are protocols needed? If so, how will they be developed and by whom? See Sidebar 2.4.

SIDEBAR 2.4: Steps to Develop and Conduct a Research Alliance

Developing an alliance with industry partners to carry out clinical research or other projects can bring benefits to not only the partners, but also the patients of an imaging facility. While the general process to set up such alliances is similar to that of other forms, the following steps can be kept in mind:

1. Prior to in-depth discussion, the appropriate legal documents should be in order (eg, nondisclosure agreement, conflict of interest disclosure form, intellectual property agreement, etc).
2. Among the first topics to discuss are the project's goals and objectives.
3. Based on the initial discussion, the type of alliance that will be most appropriate should be determined.
4. Regulations governing provider–industry relations should be thoroughly reviewed and understood by all parties, with legal advice where necessary.
5. The expected outcomes should be formally discussed and documented; these should be reviewed and validated by the appropriate parties before project implementation.
6. Once the expected outcomes are validated, the radiologists and other imaging professionals should discuss and draft the imaging protocol associated with the collaboration. This draft document is then reviewed and validated by representative experts from both partner organizations.
7. The draft imaging protocol is then tested by users with phantom images generated.
8. The phantom images and protocol instructions are reviewed by the collaborating imaging experts and vetted for expected outcomes and timelines.
9. The approved imaging protocol, outcomes, and timelines are then communicated to users.
10. User training occurs within the establish time lines.
11. The imaging protocol is implemented according to the proposed time lines.
12. When the project endpoint is reached, evaluation and analysis by the alliance partners produces final outcomes, with reporting and publication as appropriate.

4. **Marketing:** Who will be the alliance customers? Is market research needed? If so, who will carry it out and how much needs to be done before implementation? Will alliance marketing be carried out jointly?
5. **Employee compensation:** How will alliance leaders and others working on the project be compensated? If they are carrying out work for the alliance in addition to their other duties, will they receive additional compensation? What will be the status of any physicians working on the project (eg, independent contractor, partner, employee)? What performance standards will be used?
6. **Finances:** How will prices be set? What financial models will be used? Will separate budgets and accounting be needed? What reports, if any, will need to be prepared on an ongoing basis? How will partners access financial data and maintain oversight? What milestones will release pre-approved funding?
7. **Relationships:** Who will be the suppliers to the alliance? What other relationships (eg, professional organizations, business groups) will be needed and how will they be established?
8. **Regulatory oversight:** What regulations, if any, must be followed? Is accreditation or a certificate of need required (Sidebar 2.5)? If so, who will be responsible for applying and preparing for it? What quality assurance and performance measures will be used? How will ongoing compliance be ensured and by whom?

SIDEBAR 2.5: Alliances and the Certificate of Need

Before a healthcare organization can add a new service or purchase a new piece of equipment costing more than a preset limit, in 36 states (as of December 31, 2007) the organization must obtain approval from the appropriate state governmental agency. The certificate of need process aims to reduce duplication of certain high-dollar services and equipment and to maximize the healthcare dollars spent in a community by approving only those services that will improve its healthcare. In addition, the oversight agency tries to make sure the services are provided by the most appropriate healthcare provider by selecting or approving through a competitive process.

An alliance can provide a mechanism for meeting or circumventing certificate of need requirements. For example, if a state allows replacement of existing technology that has outlived its service life without demonstrating need, a facility with old equipment could ally with a partner that has been unable to demonstrate need for adding equipment. Together the partners could pool financial resources, purchase new equipment, and still meet state requirements.

The American Health Planning Association has a useful guide to the dollar thresholds and types of services regulated by each state. Before entering into an alliance, however, the state regulations currently in effect should be confirmed.

9. **Asset management:** If the alliance will own assets, how will these be shared? If a device is being developed, how will ownership of patents, the device itself, any new technology, etc, be defined?
10. **Termination:** Will the alliance have a predetermined end date? If not, how will termination be determined? How will joint assets be divided? Who will own data or other intellectual property generated by the alliance?

Many of the answers to these and similar questions will ultimately appear in the alliance business plan.

Negotiate Appropriate Agreements

Many pitfalls await those who are not diligent, open, and frank during preliminary discussions and negotiations. Even with diligence, however, most alliances will require legal consultation, and no alliance should be implemented without one or more written agreements. This section provides guidelines but does not substitute for advice from legal counsel.

Letter of Intent

Once the preparatory tasks are completed and key questions are answered, a letter of intent or memorandum of understanding should be developed. This document should include the following: (a) a summary of the key points of the alliance; (b) an acknowledgement that neither partner is now seeking an alternate partner; and (c) detailed terms under which either partner could withdraw before implementation. A time line to implementation and a confidentiality agreement may also be included. Technically speaking, a letter of intent is not considered legally binding, but in the case of substantial deals that have collapsed before a contract could be drawn up, courts have accepted the letter as contractual.[8] Therefore, both partners should carefully review the document and be willing to abide by it.

A letter of intent has a number of uses. First, it demonstrates to senior management the progress made to date and motivates them to either continue pursuing the alliance or to spend additional sums to complete market research or other tasks before implementation can take place. Second, in summarizing the key points, the document may reveal areas of disagreement that have not yet surfaced—areas that may need additional discussion or that could even stall the alliance. Third, the letter can be used to inform others about the potential alliance (eg, in preliminary discussions with a supplier with whom the alliance partners plan to work or a bank from which the partners hope to receive alliance funding). Fourth, in the case of shorter term projects such as a direct cooperation between an imaging and another hospital department, the letter of intent may be drawn up and signed in lieu of a more formal contract.

Alliance Contracts

As noted earlier, while transactions are entirely contract based, alliances allow for changing circumstances and creative problem solving. Nevertheless, most forms of alliances should have a written agreement or contract that specifies key elements, including those that must remain less than precise (eg, "cooperation among the partners"). In general, an alliance contract will deal with topics in three categories:

1. Elements of the alliance that can and should be spelled out precisely:
   - Legal structure (eg, joint venture) and governance, including the decision-making process and criteria for future key decisions
   - Scope of activities
   - Shared objectives
   - Partners' responsibilities and key resource commitments, including milestones guiding release of resources
   - Mechanisms by which costs, revenues, earnings, and risks will be shared
   - Definition of ownership of shared assets and future products or intellectual property
   - Constraints resulting from Stark or other laws, accreditation standards, or other restrictions
   - Liabilities, warranties, and other obligations to third parties (eg, landlord)
   - Mechanisms to avoid and/or solve common problems
   - Penalties for a partner's failure to perform as agreed
2. Guiding principles of the alliance, which are by nature not fully specified, such as:
   - Cooperation and trust between the partners essential to success
   - Unexpected events, changing trends, or the need to improve performance that may necessitate changes in the alliance, which the partners will work together to achieve
   - Efforts to be made to retain key personnel as long as possible to enhance performance; expectations of replacement staff members to honor their predecessors' commitments to the alliance
   - Partners' freedom to pursue other alliances beyond the scope of the present one
   - Mutually shared objectives that will guide alliance activities, but are subject to change

3. Terms guiding alliance termination, which should be clear and precise:
   - Conditions under which termination will take place, including a predetermined event (eg, project completion), a change in partner ownership, new regulations, a shift in partner's priorities, or the failure of the alliance to achieve objectives
   - Terms governing obligations to partners at termination, relating to issues such as how partners will be compensated, assets be allocated or sold, and proprietary information be allocated and protected
   - Terms resolving alliance obligations, defining how responsibilities to customers, suppliers, staff, and others will be resolved and by whom in the event of termination of the alliance

Establish Ongoing Communication Channels

Many hours will be dedicated to communications and negotiations with potential partners to establish even the simplest alliance. Once the alliance agreement has been signed, effective communication at all levels becomes even more important to the alliance success. Despite candid and open negotiations, as activities become operational, misunderstandings or disagreements may arise among alliance leaders or those assigned to implement the project. Unanticipated changes in conditions external to the alliance partners may create a need for decisive action and creative problem solving. Front-line employees may fear changes being created by the alliance, slowing its implementation. These are just a few of the scenarios that point to the need for conflict management and effective ongoing communications among all parties involved in the alliance.

Communication Between Alliance Partners

Successful alliances will use a combination of group meetings and individual conversations among alliance team members to help achieve their communication objectives. Group meetings are particularly useful for participants to receive the same information and to build consensus. Building group consensus allows participants to interact and share knowledge for successful outcomes. Given technological developments, holding a group meeting does not necessarily require time consuming and expensive travel. Using a computer-based conference calling system allows participants in diverse locations to share documents, observe body language, and participate in real-time in the discussion.

Conversations among individuals provide a rich opportunity for frankness and sharing and clarifying information. Employees at all levels of the alliance should be encouraged to engage their colleagues in discussions and to resolve operational issues. Creative problem solving and information sharing will help reach alliance objectives. When group meetings are held, opportunities for individual discussions should be incorporated. Alliance leaders should be capable of facilitating the group meetings and model positive behaviors so the group progresses toward the alliance goals.

Communication is essential especially when dealing with conflict resolution and problem solving. By avoiding hidden agendas, heated arguments, or criticism and blame, the group can work through difficult issues. When an objective is not met or performance fails to meet expectations, both parties need to focus on underlying causes and how to correct the situation. If the group can not reach consensus on the solution, it is best to avoid trying to force one side to accept a solution or to split the difference. Such tactics break down the trust needed to continue the alliance and set a pattern of evading difficult issues. Instead, the partners may need to step back, allow emotions to cool, re-examine the facts, and perhaps consider another solution on which both parties can agree. If necessary, an impartial third party could be called on to facilitate the problem solving process.

After implementation has begun, it is helpful to discuss possible scenarios that could lead to problems and how the partners will respond to them. This reduces the likelihood of conflict in the future.

Communication with Employees About an Alliance

Alliances produce changes to the status quo. The changes may be relatively small, directly affecting only a few employees (eg, direct cooperation among hospital departments), or the changes may substantially affect the way key functions are performed (eg, a joint venture to provide new services). Either way, if management does not effectively communicate with employees, even the smallest changes can result in problems.[9]

Leaders are expected to communicate to employees on a regular basis regarding information associated with the alliance.[10] The communication needs to send a clear and concise message. To facilitate a successful alliance, the communications should be crafted in a manner that emulates the leader's confidence and the employee's ability to meet expectations. The employee's anticipated reactions and emotions should be considered as messages are crafted and communicated. This exercise provides the presenter with potential responses to questions from the audience.

Whenever leaders communicate about the alliance and the changes it will bring, they aim to send the following messages[9]:

- The leader is personally committed to the alliance and whatever changes may be necessary.
- The leader recognizes that the alliance may negatively impact some employees.
- The leader is willing to listen to employee feelings about the changes.
- The leader is confident in the group's ability to work through the changes.
- The leader needs and wants employee input on ways to make the alliance work.

Ongoing communication about the alliance and potential changes should be distributed not only to employees directly involved but also to other employees and stakeholders. It is not always clear who will be affected and by how much. For example, employees who take on alliance duties are obviously affected, but their coworkers will feel the impact if they must assume neglected nonalliance duties or are unable to get nonalliance decisions in a timely fashion. Furthermore, employees not included in the communication loop may have misinformation resulting in rumors, generating unnecessary anxiety and low morale.

Communication should occur often and in a timely fashion and should provide as much accurate information as is available at the time. Delays in communicating with employees about the alliance could cause rumors resulting in false assumptions. Discussions should continue into the implementation phase to allow employees to share feelings and issues that arise once procedures are in place. Depending on the scope of the alliance it may be advisable to add communication topics to staff meeting agendas. This will provide a forum for employees to comment on the topic. Opportunities should also be available for individual employees to meet privately with their managers to share concerns or offer suggestions. It is advisable to document employee meeting discussions, especially if the information may be needed for future action.

For additional interpersonal communication techniques, see AHRA's book *Communication & Information Management in Radiology.*

Conclusion

Modern healthcare is a complex, costly enterprise. Healthcare business models have predominantly been carried out independently with sole practitioners. However, the field now relies heavily on interdependent alliances of practitioners, industry partners, vendors, and organizations. These relationships take advantage of the core competencies and creativity of the partners to achieve both business and societal objectives. Building and nurturing these relationships calls for commitment, the ability to build trust, and highly developed communication skills. Time and effort invested in forming an alliance could result in future benefits for both organizations. The growing popularity of alliances demonstrates that interdependent alliances are valuable.

References

1. Thompson AA Jr, Strickland AJ III, Gamble JE. *Crafting and Executing Strategy: The Quest for Competitive Advantage: Concepts and Cases*. NewYork, NY: McGraw-Hill; 2007.
2. Cross R. *The Hidden Power of Social Networks*. Boston, MA: Harvard Business School; 2004.
3. Making the move to a multispecialty oncology practice. *J Oncol Pract* 2008;4:68–70.
4. Sharp M, Register C, Grimes, P. *Economics of Social Issues*. New York, NY: McGraw-Hill; 2006.
5. Lewis JD. *Trusted Partners: How Companies Build Mutual Trust and Win Together*. New York, NY: The Free Press; 1999.
6. Reh FJ. Cost benefit analysis. About.com: Management. Available at: http://management.about.com/cs/money/a/CostBenefit.htm. Accessed November 23, 2008.
7. Meckin D. *Naked Finance: Business Finance Pure and Simple*. Boston, MA: Nicholas Brealey Publishing; 2007:233–241.
8. Silver JA. Letter of intent – why business people love 'em and lawyers hate 'em. Available at: http://www.letter-of-intent.com. Accessed August 20, 2009.
9. Bacal R. Introduction to the link between leadership, change management, and communication. Work911.com. Available at: http://work911.com/articles/comchan.htm. Accessed August 20, 2009.
10. Bacal R. Front and center—leadership critical to managing change. Work911.com. Available at: http://work911.com/articles/leadchange.htm. Accessed August 20, 2009.

Chapter 3

Document Processes to Ensure Service Delivery

Bonni Standley

A significant operational responsibility of an imaging management professional relates to the creation and enforcement of policies, protocols, and procedures. Clear policies and procedures that are consistently communicated and enforced have a profound positive impact on a healthcare organization. The primary purpose of these documents is to help guide staff in the pursuit of the organization's objectives and in relations with other staff within the organization. The documents are also designed to acquaint new staff with the organization and its aims, expectations, and culture, and to provide guidance to all employees for fair and consistent staff treatment. When well written, these documents describe how an organization operates, how it wants work to be carried out, why it designed the particular procedures, and what will happen for failure to comply. This chapter describes how to produce, distribute, and enforce policies and procedures that will achieve an organization's objectives.

No modern healthcare facility can or should function without policies, protocols, and procedures. These documents "help define responsibilities, maintain consistency, and are an important measure to avoid chaos in times of crisis."[1]

Policies are specified courses or methods of action based on present and future goals and can relate to activities ranging from administration to patient safety. Protocols provide a framework to guide the management of a specific disorder or clinical situation, such as the Universal Protocol to reduce medical errors incorporated into the National Patient Safety Goals of The Joint Commission. Both policies and protocols rely on procedures to provide the specific steps necessary for implementation.

While policies define specific expectations, procedures define processes. In other words, a policy provides the general direction (objective) to reach a destination (goal), whereas procedures provide the roads (methods) to accomplish the objective and goals. The procedure lays out the step-by-step pathway to achieve standardized, repeatable work patterns.

These documents are known by a variety of names, including business policies and procedures, department or desk operating procedures, standard operating procedures, quality operating procedures, or work standards.

Assess Needs for Policies and Procedures

In general, organizations use policy and procedure documents to record rules and regulations governing activities the organization considers important for its day-to-day operations. Policies and procedures covering human resource issues (eg, attendance, substance abuse), safety, patient care, productivity, and workflow are very common. The technological nature of modern imaging calls for a wide range of technical policies and procedures related to device hardware, software, image routing, quality assurance, and downtime management.

Once documented, the policies and procedures are available for everybody in the facility to refer to; these documents become the means by which decisions are made and most disputes within the organization are settled. Organizational goals and objectives cannot be achieved when consistency and fairness are lacking in the leadership decisions. Without written documentation, employees and managers lack guidance to regularly interpret routine and recurring situations.

Policies and procedures provide additional benefits that justify the effort to create them. An imaging facility with well crafted written policies is likely to be better organized and have more productive employees than one that does not.[2] Employees know what is expected and management is better able to provide the resources employees need to meet the expectations.

Well defined employee policies can settle disputes before they start and protect both the organization and its employees from confusion and the potential of litigation. A complete policy and procedure manual sets organizational standards, brings new hires up to speed more quickly, and increases overall efficiency, motivation, and professionalism. Documented policies can even be linked to profitability by reducing "downtime due to chaos or frustration"[2] and by providing a standard for measurable outcomes.

Drafting policies and procedures can be necessary for various reasons. Healthcare facilities are subject to regulatory requirements from a wide range of professional organizations and governmental agencies, including the American College of Radiology, the Centers for Medicare & Medicaid Services, and the Occupational Safety and Health Administration, and from federal, state, and local legislation,

SIDEBAR 3.1: Updating Policies and Procedures

One policy that should be incorporated into every organization's manual governs the updating process itself. An example is the provision that all existing policies would be reviewed every 2 years and revised as necessary following the procedure developed for creating and issuing policies. Some states and regulatory agencies provide guidance or have requirements for an updating process. The Joint Commission requires that if a health-care organization has an updating policy, it must be adhered to. Whenever revisions are made, the archived copy of the prior policy and the newly implemented policy need to be preserved for a period that varies by state.

ranging from the Mammography Quality Standards Act to local health laws. New or revised regulations may require additions to or revisions of existing policies and procedures to ensure compliance.

Regular review of existing policies and procedures may reveal documents that are incomplete or outdated, especially after organizational change has occurred such as installation of new technology, addition of new services, or changes in professional staff. (See Sidebar 3.1.) A review is also advisable when performance fails to meet standards; one reason for the failure may be inconsistent or incomplete policies and procedures.

Ideally, an internal audit should be performed on a regular basis to identify the need for new policies and procedures. Among the questions these audits should answer are[3]:

- Do unwritten policies exist and are they in line with the organization's objectives? Should any of these unwritten policies be codified by inclusion in the policies and procedures manual? If so, what additions/changes should be made?
- Does an issue exist that is not currently guided by a policy and procedure? If so, what are the specifics? If it involves a process, how is it currently being performed and by whom? What problems have arisen? Should changes be made in the process to improve efficiency or decrease errors? Do the outcomes meet organizational objectives?
- Do existing policies and procedures meet regulatory or other standards? If not, what needs to be done to accomplish this?

A facility will be held accountable to its written policies and procedures by patients, referring physicians, accrediting agencies, and regulators. Therefore, it is important to devise policies and procedures that (a) can be enforced and followed; (b) relate to significant work issues; and (c) contribute to workplace safety, efficiency, and patient care. While overcontrol with too many policies should be avoided, policies and procedures should be in place for issues that deal with:

- Serious consequences
- Health and safety
- Legal liability
- Licensing or regulatory requirements
- Documentation
- Accountability
- Consistency
- Clarity
- Criticality

Create Usable Documents

Policies and procedures are (or should be) documents meant to be used on a daily basis. Thus, from conceptualization to final distribution, they should be practical documents, developed with users in mind. Content should follow the 90/10 rule, that is, the policy should cover 90% of the circumstances and leave the least likely 10% as undefined.[1] Trying to cover all possible situations in a given policy or procedure is likely to make the document too long and complex, confusing users and decreasing the likelihood that it will be followed. The development process will usually have four main steps:

1. Collect background information.
2. Write a clear, concise document.
3. Evaluate the document's legal compliance.
4. Design a user-friendly document.

Collect Background Information

A variety of resources are available to create new policies and procedures. These include internal resources, external sources, and print and online publications.

One of the best ways to start the process is to survey and interview the document's end users. Asking users about any problems currently being encountered and how the users are dealing with them can provide valuable insight, and involving users in document creation will help ensure compliance once the policy is implemented.

If a series of documents is being developed (eg, for a new service), it may be useful to establish a committee representing all the user groups to provide input and review drafts. In devising procedures, users can provide detailed explanations of the current process, from which a workflow or value-stream map can be created to highlight needed changes before the procedure is standardized.

Other internal resources include existing related policies and facility publications. For hospitals or other multispecialty facilities, other departments' documents may be adapted.

A search externally for templates, best practices, and existing documents can be well worth the time and effort involved. Online resources such as Aunt Minnie, Club PACS, and MCN Healthcare offer guidelines and other resources for a fee. The Joint Commission, the Centers for Medicare & Medicaid, and other accrediting and regulatory agencies can also provide guidance for policies covered by their surveillance. Commercial software programs offer a high tech solution to drafting effective documents.

Networking among colleagues is another excellent method to solicit ideas about policies and procedures at little or no cost. Contacts may come from a variety of sources including classes, online forums, business meetings, conferences, and casual discussions. National and local imaging, healthcare, and management associations offer venues for conferring with colleagues, online forums, publications, and templates. Among the most useful are:

- ACHE: American College of Healthcare Executives
- AHRA: The Association for Medical Imaging Management
- ARMA: Administration of Records Managers Association
- ASRT: American Society of Radiologic Technologists
- BFMA: Business Forms Management Association
- RBMA: Radiology Business Managers Association
- STC: Society for Technical Communication

Many of these organizations will have journal articles and publications to assist in preparing policies and procedures. In addition, numerous books and chapters in healthcare management textbooks will offer additional resources. Among these are:

- Campbell NJ. *Writing Effective Policies and Procedures: A Step-by-Step Resource for Clear Communication*. New York: AMACOM, 1998.

- Kontaxis J. *Rapid Documentation of Policies and Procedures–The Handbook.* Hackensack, NJ: Benchmark Technologies International; 2008.
- McMillan EJ. *Model Policies and Procedures for Not-for-Profit Organizations.* 4th ed. Hoboken, NJ: John Wiley & Sons; 2008.

Write to Be Understood

For policies and procedures, a technical writing style is preferred over a narrative one, which is usually more descriptive and lengthy. Technical writing's purpose is to get a message across quickly and clearly. The shortest, clearest, strongest message comes from using normal word order, that is, subject, verb, and object. Usually, in policies and procedures, the subject will be the actor, and the verb and object will define the action required. Although it is important never to sacrifice clarity for brevity, short, simple sentences are easy to read and follow. In general, 3 to 20 words comprise a short, yet meaningful sentence.[4] Other suggestions procedure writers should try to follow include:

- Eliminate words that do not add meaning. Readers will have varying language skills and reading comprehension levels; using only the essential words will help maintain clarity and ensure compliance.
- Use words with precision. To avoid misinterpretation (and potential errors), writers should select words that say exactly what is meant.
- Create rhythm and flow by using consistency and parallelism. By organizing material in a consistent format, using consistent means of emphasis (eg, **bold to emphasize exceptions**), and presenting lists and other related material in consistent grammatical forms (eg, starting each bullet with a verb), the writer significantly increases the readability by making it easier for readers to find and follow what they need.
- Use correct grammar and usage. Following the rules improves readability and decreases misunderstandings that can result from poorly written sentences.
- Avoid negative tones. Policies and procedures should focus on what employees should do, rather than what they should not do. For example, a negative phrasing would be: "Employees may not exceed the allotted break times;" a positive phrasing would be: "Employees must observe scheduled break times under all conditions."

For additional tips to avoid writing errors and increase readability, see Sidebar 3.2.

For policies, the content should include what the rule is, why it exists, when it applies, whom it covers, enforcement, consequences, emergency contacts or references, and

SIDEBAR 3.2: Seven Cs to Avoid Procedure Writing Errors

1. Context—Actions must properly describe the activity to be performed.
2. Consistency—All references and terms must be used the same way every time, and the procedure must be written so as to ensure consistent results.
3. Completeness—There must be no gaps in information, logic, or design.
4. Control—The document and its described actions must demonstrate feedback and control.
5. Clarity—The document must be easy to read and understand.
6. Correctness—The document must be grammatically correct without spelling errors.
7. Compliance—All actions must fulfill the stated goal and must work efficiently and effectively.

Source: Bizmanualz, Inc. Seven Cs to avoid procedure writing errors. Available at: http://www.bizmanualz.com/information/2004/11/04/seven-cs-to-avoid-procedure-writing-errors.html. Accessed March 24, 2009.

how to get help or further interpretation. Procedure content includes actions, conditions for actions, alternatives, emergency procedures, consequences, warnings and cautions, help sections, examples, graphics, forms, and who is responsible.

The typical standard format includes, but is not limited to:

- A good page layout that standardizes basic information such as title, effective date, revision date, and history (ie, lists date[s] of changes to the document)
- An approval section (what staff position or committee has final authorization and approval responsibility)
- Purpose (describes objectives for writing a policy or procedure)
- Persons affected (identifies users of the document)
- Scope
- Background section
- Policy section (describes the general organizational attitude)
- Definitions (defines abbreviations, acronyms, forms, words infrequently used, and technical terms)
- Responsibilities (summarizes the roles and responsibilities of all individuals involved with the document)
- Procedures section (defines and outlines the rules, regulations, methods, timing, place, and personnel responsible for accomplishing the policy as stated in the policy section)

Some organizations use a paragraph format, while others prefer an outline format. The outline has the particular advantage of giving an immediate sense of order and logic. The material, the audience, and management guide the selection of the best format for each organization. Depending on the content, there may also be a frequently asked questions (FAQ) section and possibly some troubleshooting tips or flow charts. A sample imaging policy and procedure template is shown in Box 3.1.

Box 3.1 Sample Template for an Imaging Policy and Procedure Document

Department of Radiology

Applicable Facilities:	Department of Radiology
Effective Date:	
Revision Date:	

Purpose:

Scope:

Definitions:

Key Terms:

Policy Statements:

1.
2.
3.

Procedure Statements:

1.
2.
3.

Approved by:	
Date of Last Review:	
Next Scheduled Review Date:	
Contact Person(s):	
Resources:	
Related References:	

SIDEBAR 3.3: Policy-Related Issues That Put Organizations in Legal Jeopardy

1. Procedures used by employees that are unclear, imprecise, or poorly worded.
2. Policies or procedures that violate some law or legal precept, intentionally or unintentionally.
3. Wording that restricts the organization's ability to act; for example, a termination policy that only allows termination for cause, thus preventing the employer from firing an employee under the employment-at-will concept.
4. Written policies and procedures that are ignored or inconsistently enforced.
5. Policies or procedures that do not include descriptions of whom it applies to or what the consequences of noncompliance are.
6. Policies or procedures that are incomplete, in improper order, inaccurate, or outdated (not reflecting current practice).

Evaluate Legal Compliance

Healthcare organizations can hire, discipline, and fire employees; produce new service lines; suggest to employees what to do and how to do it; and have the right to set the rules. However, there are health and safety laws, employee and consumer rights legislation, liability laws, and contract laws that all impose certain restrictions on how healthcare organizations (and other businesses) operate. The courts hold business managers responsible for what is and could be said and done in the workplace (see Sidebar 3.3). Although the policy writer should make an effort to review the applicable laws and regulatory standards, most documents should be reviewed as well by the organization's attorneys before distribution.

One of the most fundamental considerations is the issuer's responsibility to ensure that users understand the documents. Language barriers and literacy problems may present challenges, but the writer has to make every reasonable effort to communicate clearly. Some states require that if a non–English speaking employee population comprises a specified percentage of total employees, a complete policy and procedure set must be provided in the employees' native language. To reduce literacy problems, the documents should be written at an appropriate reading level for the end users. The Americans with Disabilities Act requires employers to make reasonable accommodations to employees with disabilities, including with regard to documentation. In special circumstances (eg, an employee with dyslexia), the supervisor may want to work one-on-one with the affected employee and explain policies orally for total compliance and understanding and to avoid future legal complications.

Three types of legal violations can apply to policies and procedures: torts, negligence, and breach of implied contract. Torts are a wrongful act, one that violates a duty imposed by law and is grounds for civil action. Negligence is the failure to exercise reasonable care in instances in which care is a duty under the law. Failure to have responsible policies and procedures or the failure to communicate, follow, and enforce them can lead to charges of negligence.

Breach of implied contract involves making a promise, either orally or in writing, and then breaking it. Although policies and procedures may not be thought of as a contract, these documents state that something needs to be done in a certain way. When they do not, the injured party may file a lawsuit, claiming breach of contract. For example, if the manual describes a five step progressive disciplinary procedure to be followed leading to termination and an employee is fired without following the manual's procedure, the employee may sue as a breach of implied contract. Recognition and definition of implied contracts vary from state to state. While most states currently recognize the concept of implied contracts, court decisions and legislation may change circumstances. Thus, it is important to review all policies and procedures on a regular basis in light of current rulings, laws, and standards.

Courts have also said that contracts, expressed or implied, may carry an assumption of "good faith and fair dealing." For example, in an actual case, an employee with 18 years of service and satisfactory performance reviews was fired without adequate investigation or a hearing as provided for in the company's policies. The court ruled that dismissing an employee with a satisfactory record without legal cause violates the assumption of good faith and fair dealing implicit in a contract.[5]

Awareness of informal and/or unwritten rules that may come to govern aspects of employee work life should be noted. Although they may be informal, they can still constitute an officially sanctioned way of doing things for which courts may hold the organization responsible. For example, a manager sends an e-mail message giving directions for all staff to follow; although the staff uses the procedure for years, it does not get written into policy. If an accident occurs that can be traced to this procedure, the facility may be held liable under some circumstances.

Risks can be minimized to reduce legal exposure and provide documentation to defend actions if necessary. Courts rule based on what is said and done, so effort should be made to ensure policy and procedure content is appropriate, sufficient, and accurate and that the writing is clear, understandable, and precise. The following should be taken into consideration:

1. Word policies and procedures carefully.
2. Check the content.

3. Reserve management's right to discretionary action.
4. Preserve the right to make changes.
5. Consider the informal and unwritten rules.
6. Use and enforce the rules.

Another way to minimize risk is to include disclaimers. For example, a general disclaimer is commonly included at the front of a policy and procedure manual declaring that the manual does not constitute a contract and may be changed anytime at management's discretion. A human resources policy and procedures manual should include an employment-at-will statement (see AHRA's book *Human Resource Management in Radiology* for additional suggestions), and all policies and procedures should avoid promissory language, "weasel words" (eg, *perhaps*, *maybe*, or *almost*), and absolutes such as *always* or *never*.

Policies and procedures should also include a description of the disciplinary action or procedure for those who violate the rules and those who fail to enforce them. Further details about distributing the documents to ensure legal compliance are discussed later in this chapter.

Design with the Reader in Mind

Users of policy and procedure documents want to be able to quickly skim the page, find what they need, read and understand it, and move on to carry out their tasks. Thus, good design is very important. Are the document pages clear and easy to read or confusing and cluttered? If the latter, readers may ignore the documents; seek the information they need from another, potentially inaccurate source; or struggle through the document, with lower productivity and possibly miscommunication. As with the writing, simplicity and clarity in design are the two key ingredients to make it easy to understand and visually appealing for a reader.

Design elements that make the document friendly to readers include[4,6]:

> **Page layout**—A well-designed page considers the relationship of every element to the other elements and takes the physiology of reading into consideration. For example, putting headers or column labels on the left side of the page, and short blocks of text on the right side, takes advantage of the Western reader's tendency to start reading on the left.[4] Text chunking helps break information down into palatable bits for the reader and is accomplished by not only using short words, sentences, and paragraphs, but also by increasing the margins around the text block.

Spacing—White (or "negative") space focuses attention on the text and improves readability; this includes adequate margins (at least 1 inch) on all sides, space between lines, and additional space between sections.

Font (typeface)—Generally, fonts with serifs (the "feet" on the bottom of letters, eg, `Courier New`) are easier to read than sans serif fonts (eg, Ariel), so blocks of text should usually be presented in serif fonts. To provide visual variety, sans serif fonts can be used for short items, such as headers, titles, and even captions under illustrations. *Italic* and **bold** text formatting can be used for emphasis or as a contrast to set specific elements (eg, headers) apart from informational text.

Lists—Bulleted or numbered lists help show relationships and provide another means by which to add white space. Bullets can be used when the list items are related but random, numbers when the items are sequential.

Graphic elements—Tables, diagrams, charts, and possibly even photographs can present some information in a more meaningful way than blocks of text. They also provide variety on the page while reducing clutter by grouping related information together.

Two characteristics contribute to the effective use of these and other design elements—consistency and moderation (Box 3.2). Consistency in how elements are used provides useful signals to the reader. For example, when primary headers are printed in bold and subheaders are italic, the reader knows from page to page which items are subordinate. Consistency also helps reduce clutter that can distract and confuse the reader. On the other hand, moderation should be applied because overuse leads to ineffectiveness. For example, the effectiveness of bold type to emphasize a key point, created by its contrast with the regular type, is diminished if too much text is bold.[4,6] Overuse of bulleted or numbered lists ends up distracting and confusing the reader.

Of course, design considerations are more significant when creating an entirely new policy and procedure manual. In many instances, a document will be prepared for an existing manual for which a format (good or bad) exists and should be followed to retain consistency. When issues arise, however, that involve misunderstandings, misinterpretations, or manual disuse, design considerations should be evaluated as a possible contributing factor that could necessitate a manual redesign.

Ensure Effective Document Utilization

The time and effort needed to produce useful policies and procedures will be wasted if merely a single copy of the manual is produced to sit on a shelf in the manager's office. These documents, along with patient protocols, are (or should be)

Box 3.2 Sample Procedure for Fictitious Imaging Facility

Procedure No.: 443-14PRO
Date: January 1, 2010

Storage and Disposal of Confidential Information

1. Computer-based records

Responsible party	Step	Action
Employee	1	Use access ID and password to access confidential information as authorized and when needed.
	2	On completion of task, store data on the Imaging Facility server and close file.
	3	Delete all data on a regular basis that does not need to be stored for future use or to comply with legal requirements. If uncertain, check with supervisor before deletion.
Designated Employee	4	Back up all data at the end of each work day to the registered offsite server.
	5	Review data stored on the offsite server monthly; delete all data that are not needed for future use or legal compliance following guidelines issued by department manager.
Employee	6	If using a laptop computer offsite on which confidential data are stored or accessed, use only a computer that is encrypted and password-protected. The computer should remain in the employee's possession at all times when offsite.

2. Paper records

Responsible party	Step	Action
Employee	1	Use access ID and passcode to enter secure storage area as authorized.
	2	Obtain only those records needed for current activities and return promptly to secure storage when finished or at end of shift, whichever comes first. No records should be left in an unsecure area overnight.
	3	When disposing of any paper copies, use only secure containers designated Shred-It.
Department Manager	4	Authorize removal from Imaging Facility premises of records for patient care or legitimate business use only. Employee taking records must sign them out and back into the secure storage.
	5	Determine records to be destroyed at the end of each year, based on future use or legal compliance, and arranges for contract shredder/recycler.
Authorized Employee	6	Under manager's direction, dispose of outdated records at the end of each year using secure containers designated Shred-It.

First effective date: July 1, 2003
Last update: July 1, 2008, by jld
Last review by policy expert: July 1, 2010

the means by which the organization's mission and objectives are operationalized. Every employee should be familiar with and have access to documents relevant to his or her tasks.

Review and Responsibility

Reviewing is the final step in writing policies and procedures before implementation. An adequate review involves verification, validation, editing, proofreading, and approval. If employees were interviewed during the collection of background information, they should be asked to review the draft to help ensure that the information is accurate, understandable, and usable. The draft should be carefully reviewed for style and tone and proofread for grammatical and typographical errors. This is also the opportunity for legal review, if necessary.

In large organizations, the president or CEO will appoint a single department or committee to handle policies and procedures. This group will be empowered to manage this important responsibility, including regular updates, and draft reviews. In such cases, each department (eg, human resources) may be authorized to manage policies and procedures for its area with committee oversight and final approval. Organizations that invest in an automated policy manual management system benefit from a system feature that automatically sends out notices to the designated responsible party, usually at the typical 2 year revision sequence, when a policy should be reviewed for updates.

With or without an oversight committee, final approval authority resides with the last signature required for a given policy or procedure. It falls to the CEO/president to issue a written document designating the position(s) or individual(s) responsible for the final approving authority. Generally, a senior manager and/or the CEO/president should review all policies and procedures before distribution and implementation.

Distribution and Communication

Ensuring compliance relies on effective distribution of and communication about policies, procedures, and protocols. The first step is to identify the categories of employees and other stakeholders who are subject to the document. Many policies and procedures (eg, the human resource manual) will apply to all employees, while others will apply to one or more segments (eg, image management).

As with other steps in the process of creating policies, compliance relies on consistency in the communication process. The timing and manner of distribution, level of communication and training, and enforcement mechanisms should be specified.

As these documents are designed to comply with a legal or regulatory requirement and may become the basis for legal action, they should be distributed in one or more written forms. The employee newsletter might summarize a new facility-wide policy and refer readers to the document stored online or in a manual. Paper copies of a policy that applies to a specific group of employees could be handed out and discussed at a unit meeting. New patient care protocols could be the subject of a staff inservice training. Organizations that rely primarily on electronic communication can e-mail affected employees and attach a copy of the new policy.

New employee orientation sessions provide a mechanism for new hires to receive and review many of an organization's policies and procedures, especially those that govern human resource issues. The employees are usually asked to acknowledge in writing that they have received and read the documents. Some organizations will use online testing to evaluate the new employees' understanding of the documents.

Notifying and gaining support from managers first is important for successful implementation, especially in instances of substantial change. When new policies, procedures, and protocols involve major changes in the workplace or how work is performed, some employees may resist them. Managers who understand the policies and the needs for the changes can explain these in terms most appropriate to their subordinates. Front-line supervisors can monitor compliance closely and provide coaching when misunderstandings or further resistance arises. Early communication and ongoing education on the new material are also key to help combat any resistance to change. As noted above, if users helped write the policy, they may be more receptive to implementing it. For other suggestions of ways to avoid or reduce resistance to change, see Sidebar 3.4.

Training and Development

In many instances, distributing and communicating about policies and procedures are not enough. Employees will require proper training to develop competencies, especially when policies relate to patient care or when changes are substantial. This may occur on the job with employees demonstrating their comprehension of the new procedures, during inservice training sessions, through online testing, or with various other methods. In any format, training and development are interactive teaching tools through which management can determine whether an employee thoroughly understands the content and intent of the policy or procedure.

Accessibility and Enforcement

Enforcement is simplified when these documents are readily accessible to the affected employees, who are more likely to consult the documents if it can be done

SIDEBAR 3.4: Five Steps to Deliver Unpopular Policies and Procedures

Delivering unpopular news always demands a manager's best communication skills and this is especially true when policies will involve substantial workplace changes or are otherwise unpopular with employees. The following steps can be used to reduce employee fear and help smooth the process:

1. **Involve**—Key staff members should be consulted before, during, and after drafting the document. Whenever possible, the users' interests should be put first. Before full implementation an employee focus group can test the draft to poke holes in it and find any unforeseen loopholes.
2. **Explain**—The reasons for the policy should be explained thoroughly, with data and facts to establish the background. The manager should be honest and avoid delaying, which will encourage rumors and gossip.
3. **Listen**—Employees should have multiple sessions to express their fears, complaints, and concerns. It may be useful to create a complaint system (if one does not exist) and be prepared to meet one on one.
4. **Enforce**—Advance notice of the policy's implementation should be given and all employees should have the training necessary to successfully comply with it. While flexibility is advisable during the initial implementation phase, the manager should make clear that failure to comply is not an option. Policy enforcement should be consistent.
5. **Evaluate**—Compliance should be closely monitored. After a period of adjustment, the implementation process should be reviewed and any changes noted that should be made when the next policy must be implemented.

quickly and without disrupting workflow. Accessibility relates to both the location of the physical document and to a document structure that allows users to quickly find the information sought. In addition to design elements, document components such as a table of contents (Box 3.3), lists of illustrations and forms, an introduction detailing the purpose and scope, a glossary, an appendix, and an index all contribute to the user's ability to efficiently find the needed information.

With regard to the physical document, many healthcare organizations now store their policies, procedures, and protocols on the facilities' server in a password-protected intranet depository accessible to employees and other stakeholders. This eliminates the tedious process of inserting updates into manuals located throughout the facility. Instead, when there is a substantial change, an electronic update alert is sent to the employees who are affected. The e-mail can summarize the changes and refer the employee to the correct location on the server or the full revised document can be attached to the e-mail. An electronic receipt can acknowledge that each employee has received and opened the e-mail, for compliance purposes. However, because opening an e-mail does not guarantee a full

Box 3.3 Sample Table of Contents for a Policy and Procedure Manual

Introduction
Acknowledgments

Administration and Finance
Human Resources
Equipment
Film File Management
General Safety
Radiation Safety
Infection Control
Patient Care
Results Reporting
Cardiac Catheterization
Interventional Radiology
Magnetic Resonance Imaging
Mammography
Nuclear Medicine

Resources
Web Sites

reading or understanding of the document, additional communication should be carried out.

Of course, smaller facilities may want to continue to use paper manuals because employees often find the process easier and faster to take a book off a shelf than to access the appropriate server location. Copies should be widely available, with a record made of the location of each copy, so when revisions are needed, all manuals can be quickly found and updated.

For legal purposes, a complete set of policies, procedures, and protocols that includes all previous versions should be retained in a safe location. As nearly all policy and procedure manuals will have begun as paper copies (before the computer age), many facilities will keep a complete paper set for this purpose. Alternatively, facilities that are entirely electronic can scan historical paper versions onto a computer, track changes on more recent electronic versions, and retain this set on the server as a locked master that cannot be overwritten. The ongoing process of review and revision would include the final step of adding the new documents to this master set. State regulations governing the number of years these master sets must be kept vary by state, but a 7 year requirement is common.

Among the policies and procedures should be one or more governing enforcement of all such documents, which describes the person responsible for determining compliance, the penalties for failing to comply, and any appeal process. As with other policies, those governing enforcement should be consistently applied to avoid any perception of unfairness, to encourage compliance with all policies, and to reduce the potential for employee lawsuits.

Conclusion

A well crafted set of policies, protocols, and procedures is one of the most important sets of operational documents in a healthcare organization. They tangibly demonstrate an organization's professionalism to accrediting and regulatory agencies. These documents guide employees in carrying out their daily tasks and contribute to communicating the organization's mission and values. When these documents are followed, they ensure consistent and superior patient care, contribute to high employee morale, and help bring about financial stability and soundness.

References

1. Knepper D. PACS policies and procedures. *Radiol Manage.* 2007;29(2):16-21.
2. Mason S. Promoting the need for P&P documentation. In: Mason S, Maggiani R, Margulies J, Robinson RE. Policy and procedure communication and the lone writer. Panel presented at: 2002 Annual Conference, Society for Technical Communication. Available at: http://www.stc.org/ConfProceed/2002/PDFs/STC49-00056.pdf. Accessed September 4, 2009.
3. Kroken P, Richardson E, Stockburger W, eds. *Communication & Information Mangement in Radiology.* Sudbury, MA: American Healthcare Radiology Administrators; 2007;135.
4. Fleming JR. Writing clear policies and procedures with Playscript. Presented at: 1999 Annual Conference, Society for Technical Communication. Available at: http://www.stc.org/ConfProceed/1999/PDFs/stc-37.pdf. Accessed September 4, 2009.
5. *Cleary v American Airlines,* 111 Cal App 3d 443, 168 Cal Rptr 722 (1980).
6. Williams R. *The Non-Designer's Design Book.* Berkeley, CA: Peachpit Press; 1994.

Chapter 4

Develop Examination Protocols and Evaluate Results

Douglas Cathon and Janice Eurton

The importance of medical imaging in patient care management continues to grow. Not only is medical imaging an important method of diagnosis, it also plays an increasingly important role in patient care through the use of coordinated treatment plans. Diagnostic and therapeutic medical imaging benefits the patient through rapid and precise disease management, fewer side effects, and improved outcomes. In addition, medical imaging benefits the healthcare system through improved efficiency and more cost-effective solutions. Developing protocols is critical to establishing effective, streamlined operations ensuring quality and safety for both the employee and the patient.

The use of standard protocols in imaging has many benefits to the facility and its customers. Protocols ensure the accuracy of procedures and afford the patient increased safety measures by the uniform completion of exams each time they are performed. Technologists have standards to follow and any deviation from these can be addressed through established measures that have been determined in advance and documented. The use of protocols can be a method to increase productivity by creating a more efficient and consistently performing department—from the scheduling process through the conclusion of procedures—and removing obstacles to completing procedures as scheduled. The effective use of protocols allows more patient volume with less manpower due to avoidance of undue delays (eg, trying to contact the radiologists and/or ordering physicians for clarification of orders, or determining the appropriateness of ordered procedures).

Specific protocols that include screening tools must be developed and presented to all parties involved with the imaging process. Following an established plan enables referring physicians to answer specific questions in relation to clinical scenarios and individual patients, such as: Is imaging indicated? Will imaging change the diagnosis? Will the imaging report change the patient's care management?

Unnecessary or inappropriate exams expose the patient to risk without additional benefit and can deter the effective allocation of resources. The wrong choice of a test may lead to a delay in diagnosis and could result in inappropriate care to the patient. To reduce inappropriate ordering of diagnostic imaging examinations, protocols need to include both the referring physicians and the providers of the imaging services. See Box 4.1 for a sample policy on appropriate indications for a procedure.

Box 4.1 Sample Policy on Appropriate Indications for Procedure

<table>
<tr><td>ABC Hospital</td><td>Page 1 of 1</td><td>RVS</td><td>RVW</td></tr>
<tr><td rowspan="2">NAME OF POLICY:
Appropriate Indications for Procedure</td><td>POLICY #:</td><td rowspan="4">8/07</td><td rowspan="4">2/05
2/08</td></tr>
<tr><td>EFFECTIVE DATE: 7/2003</td></tr>
<tr><td>AREA: Patient Care</td><td>WRITTEN BY:</td></tr>
<tr><td>DEPARTMENT:
Medical Imaging</td><td>APPROVED BY:
Medical Imaging Medical Director</td></tr>
</table>

<table>
<tr><td colspan="2">POLICY STATEMENT:
To ensure appropriate indications are documented prior to the performance of a medical imaging study.</td></tr>
<tr><td>PERSONS AFFECTED:</td><td>PROCEDURES:</td></tr>
<tr><td>■ CT Technologist
■ MRI Technologist
■ Nuclear Medicine Technologist
■ Radiographer
■ Sonographer</td><td>1. Will compare patient's symptoms or diagnosis with the procedure requested in the chart or on the patient's order prior to performing the procedure.
2. Will contact the nursing floor, patient's physician, and/or physician's office if appropriate indications for the study are not documented.
3. Will return patient to nursing floor if unable to clarify indications for procedure for an inpatient.
4. Will complete a Telephone/Verbal Order sheet if physician is contacted and appropriate indications are clarified.
5. Will contact the physician's office and request a new order be faxed to the hospital with the correct procedure and/or appropriate diagnosis for an outpatient.
6. Will discuss with outpatient the reasons why the procedure cannot be performed if physician or physician's office cannot be contacted for correct procedure and/or appropriate diagnosis.</td></tr>
</table>

All imaging resources have peaks and valleys in terms of utilization. In order to use time, people, and equipment effectively, operational workflows need to be analyzed. Considerations might be:

- When are the facility's peak times?
- What is the maximum capacity of the equipment and personnel?
- Are supplies being used appropriately and are they readily available?
- How proficient are imaging personnel in performing their duties? Are these duties documented in a competency?

Answers to these questions can be incorporated into the standardized protocols, leading to a more efficient and productive imaging facility in which daily routine becomes more streamlined and manageable, and the patient is assured of appropriate imaging services.

Obtaining Radiologist Buy-In

Developing protocols benefits the radiologists, as it lessens the amount of work they do, reduces the risk of errors, provides a strong basis for teaching, and results in timely and accurate diagnostic interpretations. Often radiologists are reluctant to participate in developing protocols because they cannot come to agreement on unified standards to obtain and present imaging procedures for review. Some may fear if they are not in complete agreement with established protocols it could adversely affect them during litigation. It is imperative the radiologists are brought to a consensus to enable the facility to move forward with building appropriate protocols to provide patients and their physicians with quality imaging examinations.

The radiologist has the responsibility to ensure radiation exposure to patients and staff is the minimum necessary to achieve results, according to ALARA (as low as reasonably achievable) principles. The medical director or chairman of the imaging facility must insist that all radiologists act as gatekeepers. Requests should be reviewed to ensure appropriate clinical information matches the examination requested by the referring physician. In addition, the radiologist must consider the best possible scanning scenario which will provide the most accurate information with least amount of exposure and discomfort to the patient. This is accomplished through the utilization of protocols which reduce wait times and improve throughput, yet maintain a high quality diagnostic image. Also, see Boxes 4.2 and 4.3 for an example of a radiologist peer review process that would satisfy the American College of Radiology (ACR) modality accreditation requirements.

Box 4.2 Radiologist Peer Review Process

1. Imaging studies will be randomly selected for peer review; all modalities will be reviewed.
2. A peer review form will be stapled to the report from the prior study selected for review.
3. As you are reviewing the current study, please peer review the prior study.
4. If you agree with the prior interpretation, check the first box for "peer rating 1."
5. If you don't agree with the prior interpretation, check the appropriate box.
6. Place the completed form with report into the locked boxed in your reading station marked "CONFIDENTIAL".
7. The information from the peer review forms will be collated and reported to the Quality Improvement Committee (QIC). Basic information will be kept in a format that will satisfy the ACR modality accreditation requirements.
8. Following the basic data gathering, the peer review sheets will be destroyed.
9. Studies that have been rated as a "3" or "4", will be given to Dr. X for the Internal Peer Review Committee to review.
10. Any comments written on the peer review sheet will be typed and given to the committee for their review. The name of the radiologist that over read the study will be withheld.
11. The Internal Peer Review Committee shall determine the final rating and report any action taken back to the QIC.
12. Below is the sample report to QIC.

Radiology Summary	General	CT	MR	US	Nuc Med	Other	Sum
Peer rating 1							
Peer rating 2							
Peer rating 3							
Peer rating 4							
Total cases reviewed							

The use of protocols allows for the maintenance of workflow and continuity of service when staff—medical or nonmedical—leave the facility. Additionally, a check and balance review system should be developed and documented to assure personnel development is in place and the staff are adhering to the established protocols.

Best Practices

Standardized protocol development allows providers to design a best practice for each situation. These standards should be built on evidence-based practice, service expectations, and the mission and vision of the organization. Input from the medical director, department administrator, and the technologists concerning the

Box 4.3 Peer Review Worksheet

This study has been randomly selected for PEER REVIEW today.

Study:

The 4 point review classification system is the same as the American College of Radiology's (ACR) RADPEER system. Rating Scale:

- ☐ 1 = Concur with interpretation
- ☐ 2 = Difficult diagnosis, not ordinarily expected to be made

---

- ☐ 3 = Diagnosis should be made most of the time
- ☐ 4 = Diagnosis should be made most of the time—misinterpretation of findings

Rating of 3 or 4 will be reviewed by the Radiologists Internal Peer Review Committee. Please note your comments or concerns below:

____

Signature / Peer Reviewer

When finished, please place this form and report in the locked "confidential" box in your reading area.

capabilities of the equipment and staff; consideration of patient acuity levels; and analysis of case mix will prove to be valuable tools in creating the development of protocols.

There is a plethora of information online relating to protocol development and usage, available from the following sources:

- ACR Appropriateness Criteria
- American College of Cardiology (ACC) Appropriateness Criteria
- American Imaging Management (AIM)
- Society of Interventional Radiology (SIR)
- Society of Nuclear Medicine (SNM)
- Centers for Medicare and Medicaid Services (CMS)

Protocol workflow is very dependent on size and structure of the facility. In order to relieve the stress of paperwork, a first step is to design a protocol manual and post the protocol literature in a visual folder by each workstation. This protocol manual should include all aspects of protocol, including the pre and post aspects of an exam. Protocol sheets can be designed with various choices so that a radiologist can simply check off the necessary boxes. See Box. 4.4 for an example of a protocol for a lower extremity venous ultrasound.

A radiology information system (RIS) allows for the radiologist to receive the requisition on a worklist as soon as it is placed, electronically select the appropriate protocol, and send the request to the technologist's worklist of exams to perform. However, the downside to this technology is that even though it expedites procedures, protocols still need to be standardized so that no matter who receives the requisition, the same selection comes to the technologist performing the exam. Special changes can be made based on specific patient clinical information, but the majority of the exams reviewed will have the same selection of images.

A major challenge is staying compliant with technology changes. Identify what changes can be made in the workflow to use speed, control exposure, and make sure that resources are used appropriately. Innovations in protocol writing are also moving forward whereby the radiologist who receives the request on his worklist can check the protocol and send that information to a specific piece of equipment. The information will then be uploaded and logged. When the patient name is entered, the protocol will appear and the technologist can go immediately to scanning the patient. Everyone wants to follow the "best practices" methodology, but it has to be accomplished within the organizational structure.

Modality Specific Considerations

An imaging facility comprises multiple departments, each utilizing its own areas of expertise and equipment. Each department should be analyzed to determine pertinent protocols that best suit the workflow and radiologist's needs to ensure high-quality images are obtained on an ongoing basis.

General Diagnostic Imaging

General radiographic procedures are no less important than any other specialty area of imaging. In the age of computed and digital radiography (CR and DR), strict protocols must be put into place assuring patients are receiving quality examinations

Box 4.4 Sample Protocol

ABC HOSPITAL
DIAGNOSTIC IMAGING

Lower Extremity Venous Ultrasound

Approved Date: 10/03/03 Revised 3/3/05
Reviewed 9/07, 10/08

PURPOSE

To rule out or identify thrombosis in the veins of the legs; to identify the exact location and extent of the thrombus; to allow qualitative analysis of its characteristics

INDICATIONS

Leg pain of questionable etiology; tight, swollen leg; tenderness in the leg; feeling of heaviness in the leg; discoloration of the leg; question of pulmonary embolism; surveillance before or after surgery or other high-risk event; chronic leg ulcers or stasis color changes in the leg; varicose veins (preoperative scan)

CONTRAINDICATIONS AND LIMITATIONS

Site trauma such as open wounds over the scan area; severe obesity; severe leg edema; patients who cannot be adequately positioned; uncooperative patients or patient refusal

EQUIPMENT

High-resolution ultrasound system with color and spectral Doppler capabilities; transducers with frequencies in the 2- to 10-MHz range; stretcher that can produce a reverse Trendelenburg's position

PATIENT PREPARATION & HISTORY

The sonographer introduces him/herself and explains the exam to the patient. Document the patient's symptoms and relevant medical history on the venous worksheet. The patient changes into a gown and disrobes from the waist down. The patient is positioned on the stretcher in a supine position. On the leg being examined, the hip is slightly rotated externally and the knee slightly bent. The bed or table is placed in a reverse Trendelenburg's position (head elevated about 10° to 20°). The room should be warm. If the room is cool and temperature cannot be regulated, warm the patient by using heated blankets or other measures.

STUDY PROTOCOL

If a unilateral study, always document the contralateral CFV with a spectral Doppler waveform.

Short axis 2D with compression on a dual image:

1. CFV with the common femoral artery laterally.
2. CFV with the GSV medially (saphenofemoral junction).
3. An image of the first 2–3 in. of the greater saphenous vein.
4. Profunda (deep) femoral and SFV just below their junction.
5. SFV with the superficial femoral artery for proximal SFV.
6. Mid thigh for SFV.
7. Distal thigh for distal SFV *or* the distal SFV may be taken at the back of the knee when doing the popliteal vein.
8. Popliteal vein with popliteal artery.
9. Posterior tibial at the distal calf.
10. Posterior tibial at the mid calf.
11. Peroneal at the mid calf.
12. Posterior tibial/peroneal trunk at proximal calf.

Short axis color Doppler evaluation to demonstrate wall-to-wall flow:

Color image of the:

- CFV
- CFV with GSV
- SFV and PFV
- SFV mid thigh
- Popliteal vein

Long axis spectral Doppler evaluation:

- CFV with distal augmentation from above the knee and below the knee.
- Popliteal with distal augmentation.

Annotate images by identification of vessel and location (eg, proximal, mid, or distal thigh or lower leg). *Do not identify veins as proximal, mid, or distal.*

Additional images may be obtained as necessary to document pathology.

DOCUMENTATION

The Lower Extremity Venous Worksheet will be completed pre-exam to include physician's indication for exam, patient's history, risk factors, and other pertinent information. Post-exam information will be written on the worksheet and scanned into RIS.

INTERPRETATION

Criteria for patency of all veins:

1. Complete coaptability of the vein walls with the ultrasound transducer.
2. Absence of intraluminal thrombus discerned from B-mode image in transverse and longitudinal planes.
3. Normal venous Doppler (spectral or color) signals of spontaneity, phasicity, and augmentation.
4. Visualization of blood flow throughout the lumen with color Doppler.

Criteria for acute venous thrombosis:

1. Lack of complete compressibility of vein.
2. Visualization of intraluminal thrombus with complete or partial obstruction of the vein lumen.
3. Distention of the vein compared to the adjacent artery.
4. Free floating, partially attached thrombus.
5. Abnormal venous Doppler signals (ie, continuous non-phasic flow, reduced or absent flow with distal augmentation, or no signal).
6. Continuous, non-phasic flow in a CFV unilaterally, with phasic flow in the contralateral CFV suggests an iliac vein outflow obstruction (ie, DVT or extrinsic compression).

Criteria for an acute versus chronic DVT:

If a patient is symptomatic for a DVT and the thrombus is of uncertain chronicity, the thrombus should be considered acute unless it can be clearly demonstrated to be chronic.

Criteria for chronic DVT:

1. Thrombus has increased echogenicity.
2. Vein is contracted and is often the same size or smaller than the adjacent artery. In very old DVT, the vein may be so contracted that it may not be apparent on the ultrasound image.
3. Large collateral veins are often present.
4. Recanalization with partial lumen restoration. Residual, fibrous bands are often seen following recanalization.
5. Vein walls may be thickened.
6. Calcium deposits may be observed within old thrombus.

REPORTING

An interventional radiologist interprets all venous ultrasound studies. When an interventional radiologist is not available, a non-interventional radiologist may give a preliminary report for the exam. The interventional radiologist will give the final interpretation of the study as soon as available.

Normal Exam: If an inpatient, completion of the exam is documented in the chart in the Physician Progress Notes. If an outpatient, the patient may go home and be instructed to await subsequent instructions from the referring physician.

Abnormal Exam: If the results are positive, the interventional radiologist or designee notifies the referring physician of the results. If an inpatient, completion of the exam is documented in the chart on the Physician Progress Notes. If an outpatient, the patient's referring physician is contacted before the patient leaves the facility.

The final report of the examination will include the following:

1. Patient's name, date, exam performed, history and indications for the study.
2. Body of report (findings).

I. Unilateral Exam
   A. Identify limb being examined and proximal/distal extent of interrogation
      - Comment on compressibility
      - Gray-scale findings (presence and location of thrombus, if present), color and spectral Doppler findings when appropriate, including identification of phasic flow and augmentation
      - If thrombus is seen, identify if acute or chronic

   B. Comment on spectral waveform of contralateral vein

II. Bilateral Exam
   A. Right Side
      - Identify limb being examined and proximal/distal extent of interrogation
      - Comment on compressibility
      - Gray-scale findings (presence and location of thrombus, if present), color and spectral Doppler findings when appropriate, including identification of phasic flow and augmentation
      - If thrombus is seen, identify if acute or chronic

   B. Left Side
      - Identify limb being examined and proximal/distal extent of interrogation
      - Comment on compressibility
      - Gray-scale findings (presence and location of thrombus, if present), color and spectral Doppler findings when appropriate, including identification of phasic flow and augmentation
      - If thrombus is seen, identify if acute or chronic

3. Comments about limitations of the study or deviations from usual interpretive criteria.
4. Comparison with results of prior studies.
5. Impression or conclusion—Location of thrombus and identification as acute or chronic.

CLEANING AND CARE OF EQUIPMENT

Before each exam the transducer is cleaned with disinfectant solution.

REFERENCES

1. Zweibel WJ. *Introduction to Vascular Ultrasonography*. 5th ed. Philadelphia, PA: Elsevier, Inc.; 2005.
2. Daigle RJ. *Techniques in Noninvasive Vascular Diagnosis*. 2nd ed. Littleton, CO: Summer Publishing; 2002.
3. Talbot SR, Oliver MA. *Techniques of Venous Imaging*. Pasadena, CA: Appleton Davies, Inc.; 1992.
4. American College of Radiology. ACR practice guideline for the performance of peripheral venous ultrasound examination. Reston, VA: ACR; 2006.

with minimal radiation exposure. Parameters should be maintained in regards to exposure techniques and settings of equipment, especially in the area of portable radiography where technologists may choose to overexpose the patient in hopes of avoiding a repeat image.

Proper shielding of all patients should be addressed, especially children and women who are pregnant or of childbearing age. Additionally, technologists should adhere to protocols incorporating radiation safety in the operating suite, ensuring all staff members and physicians are protected from radiation exposure at all times.

CT Scan

Computed tomography (CT) scans have become a pivotal diagnostic tool in aiding in the treatment of the patient. The basic information provided to the CT department is unchanged in that the order needs to validate the medical necessity of the exam. Like many imaging studies, CT has its own variables such as:

- Specific exams require the use of contrast media; therefore, prior to having contrast-related studies a patient may need to have a BUN and/or creatinine level lab test done. The results must be within specific parameters to allow for the contrast study to be done safely without harm to the renal system.
- A contrast risk assessment form is completed by asking the patient specific health questions.
- The signs/symptoms or diagnosis given by the ordering physician should be reviewed by the radiologist or technologist to ensure the appropriate exam has been ordered and any questions clarified with either the radiologist or the ordering physician before completing the requested examination.

Because of the tremendous amount of information that can be acquired with new multislice scanners, standardized protocols must be in place. This allows any radiologist viewing the study to see the same anatomical information on each case. Protocols may include but are not limited to:

- Type and amount of contrast used
- Number and thickness of images sliced
- Return on investment (ROI) measurements
- Breath holds or breathing assistance from the patient
- The correct use of contrast media according to examination ordered

To support the realm of CT scanning and reduce possible risk factors, the following policies must be in place:

- Contrast nephrotoxicity risk screening
- Contrast extravasation reporting
- Contrast reaction and initial management of reactions
- Contrast reaction risk screening

- Critical results reporting
- Contrast storage
- Discharge instructions post-contrast (facility dependent)

The above criteria should be developed following the established standards of practice relevant to the facility's practice guidelines.

Fluoroscopic Studies

Fluoroscopy is a continuous beam X-ray used to produce a video image of a particular body part. This method of imaging is used in interventional procedures for guiding placement of catheters, wires, or stents. It is also used in assessment of stomach and bowel movement, many operative procedures, and detection of obstructions in an airway or blood vessel.

Radiation safety is a constant concern when utilizing fluoroscopy. One area of particular concern is the amount of time the fluoroscopic unit is used on a patient. ALARA principles should be strictly adhered to when performing fluoroscopy and the standardization of fluoroscopy studies allows for the patient and staff to receive a minimal amount of radiation.

Though updated technology has allowed for the improvement of equipment design and enhancements which reduce the amount of radiation, ACR now requires reporting of the exposure time in the patient's final report.[1] This calls for the imaging facility, either through a manual process or electronically through the RIS, to provide the radiologist with the actual amount of fluoroscopy time which the radiologist will document in the final interpretation.

Interventional Radiology/Special Procedures

Interventional imaging and interventional neuroradiology are clinical subspecialties of radiology focused on minimally invasive, image guided procedures for numerous diseases and pathology. Interventional imaging begins with the initial consultation, often involving steps of therapeutic intervention and continuing to eventual resolution of the clinical problem or establishment of a managed care plan.

Established protocols are especially important in the interventional lab. There is a need for monitoring patients closely for adverse reactions and their treatment to have more specific charting guidelines. A current history and physical is now a requirement prior to beginning these procedures as well as adherence to universal protocols (as required by The Joint Commission) to initiate a time-out prior to site and procedure identification. Interventional procedures are not only diagnostic, but therapeutic in nature and are treated as carefully as procedures performed in the operating room.

The use of protocols in the interventional lab ensures the procedure is performed in the same manner from beginning to end every time on every patient.

Mammography

Periodic mammography screening of age appropriate asymptomatic women is vital in the early detection of breast cancer. Mammography, long held as the gold standard in breast imaging, is now accompanied by ultrasound and more recently breast MRI in the treatment and detection of breast disease.

It is essential mammography be performed and interpreted with the highest quality standards and protocols possible. Digital mammography allows for the most detailed images with the least amount of radiation; affords the radiologist the ability to focus on areas of concern through various enhancement tools without additional images having to be obtained; and saves the patient unnecessary radiation. Computer-aided detection (CAD) is an additional tool available to the radiologist to have the images over read by the computer software, drawing attention to possible areas of concern the naked eye may have missed.

All mammography must be performed in accordance with the Mammography Quality Standards Act (MQSA) final rule as published by the US Food and Drug Administration (FDA). Strict protocols and compliance are mandated through annual inspections by authorized agencies and periodic recertification of the facility by the FDA.

Magnetic Resonance Imaging

Magnetic resonance imaging (MRI) is performed by the use of an extremely strong magnetic field. Though MRI is not a radiation-based procedure, there are major concerns for both employee and patient safety. Protocols should be in place to assure all individuals working within the MRI environment are documented to have successfully completed at least one initial MRI safety lecture or safety video and to show evidence of annual competency as well.

There should be a definitive division of personnel. Level 1 comprises basic MR safety and is intended for personnel not actually working inside the magnetic field, but who may have limited exposure to the room. Level 2 personnel need more extensive training that includes aspects of MR safety associated with working inside the magnetic field. The following are important aspects relating to MRI protocols:

- Device/object screening: There should be access to a handheld magnet to test equipment in the environment and individuals who may not have been previously screened. All portable metallic or partially metallic devices must be documented as being made of a nonferromagnetic substance.

- Procedures: If the patient has a cardiac pacemaker, epicardial pacer wire, or any other type of muscle or nerve stimulator, the patient should not be scanned unless it known the device is MRI compatible. Scans should not be performed if the following devices have not successfully passed device/object screening:
  - Intracranial aneurysm clips
  - Arteriovenous malformation clips
  - Prosthetic eyes
  - Metallic fragments in the eye
  - Ear implants

Additionally, patients with permanent eyeliner or certain types of tattoos should not be scanned as the dyes may become hot and cause burns to the patient. The single most important aspect to performing an MRI exam is the screening process. Careful design and strict adherence to safety protocols should be a major focus of every MRI department.

See Box 4.5 for a sample MRI safety form, showing documentation of second reviewer in nonemergent cases.

Nuclear Medicine/Nuclear Cardiology

Nuclear medicine is a subspecialty of medical imaging in which images are obtained after injection of a small dose of a radiopharmaceutical to diagnose or treat a variety of diseases, including but not limited to cancer, heart disease, and certain other abnormalities. These tests are noninvasive and usually painless. Prior to any nuclear scan being performed, the radiologist or cardiologist may review the patient's clinical and historical information to determine the medical necessity of the exam being ordered and make recommendations to the ordering physician if changes are to be made according to established department protocols.

There are risks associated with nuclear imaging and nuclear cardiac imaging which should be recognized and protocols put in place to reduce danger to both patient and employee.

General Nuclear Imaging

Because the doses of radioactive tracer are small, the risk of significant radiation exposure is low. However, strict safety protocols should be followed at all times and are a requirement of the Nuclear Regulatory Commission (NRC). Allergic reactions

Box 4.5 Sample MRI Safety Form

DEPARTMENT OF RADIOLOGY
MRI SAFETY SCREENING SHEET

⚠ **WARNING:** Certain implants, devices, or objects may be hazardous to you and/or may interfere with the MR procedure (ie, MRI or MR Angiography [MRA]). **Do not enter** the MR system room or MR environment if you have any question or concern regarding an implant, device, or object. Consult the MRI technologist or radiologist BEFORE entering the MR system room. **The MR system magnet is ALWAYS on.**

Please indicate if you have any of the following:

NO	YES	
□	□	Cardiac pacemaker or implanted cardiac defibrillator (ICD)
□	□	Coronary or cardiac stent
□	□	Aneurysm clip(s)
□	□	Neurostimulator (TENS)
□	□	Cochlear, otologic, or ear implant
□	□	Insulin or infusion pump
□	□	Any implanted catheter (Infusaport, Swan-Ganz, etc)
□	□	Shrapnel, BB, gunshot, or bullet
□	□	Any type of intravascular coil, filter, or stent (IVC filter, coronary stent)
□	□	Heart valve prosthesis or replacement
□	□	Penile implant or prosthesis
□	□	Eye implant or prosthesis
□	□	Surgical clips, staples, or metallic sutures
□	□	Shunt (spinal or intraventricular)
□	□	Artificial limb or joint replacement
□	□	Intrauterine device (IUD) or diaphragm
□	□	Any implanted orthopedic device (pins, screws, nails, plates)
□	□	Any metal shavings or shards in your eyes (are you a metal worker?)
□	□	Medication patch (nicotine, nitroglycerine, pain) (remove before MRI)
□	□	Tattoo or permanent makeup
□	□	Body piercing jewelry (remove before MRI)
□	□	Dentures or partial plates (remove before MRI)
□	□	Hearing aid (remove before MRI)
□	□	Breathing problem
□	□	Motion disorder
□	□	Claustrophobia

Please mark on the figure(s) below the locations of any implant or metal inside of or on your body.

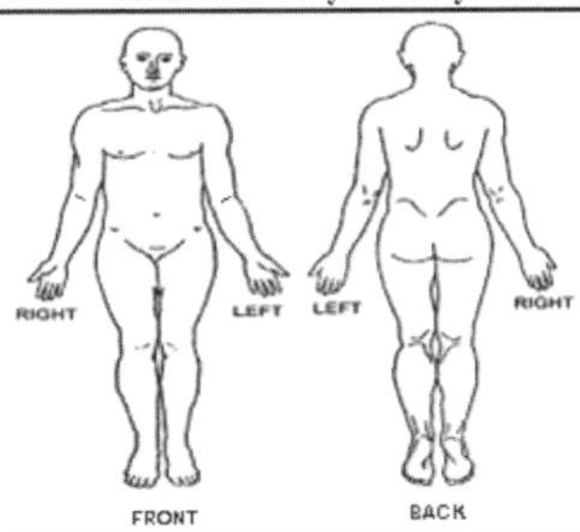

⚠ **IMPORTANT INSTRUCTIONS**

Before entering the MR environment or room, you must remove all metallic objects including hearing aids, dentures, partial plates, keys, beeper, cell phone, eyeglasses, hair pins, barrettes, jewelry, body piercing jewelry, watch, safety pins, paperclips, money clip, credit cards, bank cards, magnetic strip cards, coins, pens, pocket knife, nail clipper, tools, clothing with metal fasteners, and clothing with metallic threads.

NOTE: You may be advised or required to wear earplugs or other hearing protection during the MRI procedure to prevent possible problems or hazards related to loud noise.

I attest that the above information is correct to the best of my knowledge. I have read and understand the contents of this form and had the opportunity to ask questions regarding the information on this form and regarding the MR procedure that I am about to have done.

Patient/Parent/Guardian Signature ____________ Relationship ____________ Date ____________

Form Completed By: □ Patient □ Relative □ Nurse (Sign Below – 1st Review) □ Othe ____________

Healthcare Staff Signature (1st Review) ____________ Technologist Signature (2nd Review) ____________ Date ____________

AFFIX PATIENT LABEL

Form #734-0001 / Rev. 03-09

Source: Vaughan Regional Medical Center, Selma, AL. Used with permission.

may occur but are extremely rare and are usually mild. Nevertheless, department protocol for any type of reaction should be followed. There should be strict concern for women who may be pregnant or breastfeeding. Protocols should be developed that include the contact made with the ordering physician concerning potential risks before proceeding with the requested procedure.

Nuclear Cardiology

Nuclear cardiology involves patients with known or suspected risk of cardiac disease. During a procedure, it is possible the patient could experience chest pain or an adverse cardiac event during the exercise portion of the procedure or when drugs are given for the stress test. If life-threatening cardiac disease is suspected because of test findings, there may be an immediate need for cardiovascular intervention. Protocols should be in place to address these issues and any other adverse events, ensuring correct measures are taken in a timely fashion to assist the patient.

Positron Emission Tomography/Computed Tomography

Since its introduction in 1998, dual-modality positron emission tomography/computed tomography (PET/CT) imaging has received great attention in the medical community. A whole-body survey is the standard mode of acquisition. The CT images are used for anatomic reference of the tracer uptake patterns imaged in PET, as well as for attenuation correction of the PET data. The routine use of CT-based attenuation correction and user preferences for the quality and type of the CT examination has led to the introduction of different PET/CT scanning protocols.

Two general approaches to PET/CT imaging can be distinguished today. One uses CT as a fast transmission source with little additional information for anatomic labeling. The other uses CT as a fast transmission source as well as a state-of-the-art diagnostic tool to maximize image quality using optimal acquisition parameters together with oral and intravenous contrast agents. Variations of these approaches share common concerns about image artifacts that result from mismatches in respiration and patient positioning between the CT and PET examinations.

Protocol requirements for the more complex radiologic PET/CT scenario also include alternative contrast application schemes or modifications to the attenuation correction procedure to handle CT contrast agents appropriately.[2]

Ultrasound

Ultrasound images are acquired via sound waves to evaluate various internal organs and anatomy for disease or abnormalities as well as determine fetal health in utero. Ultrasound image acquisition is extremely operator dependent. Only well qualified sonographers should be performing sonography procedures.

A major consideration for ultrasound is having protocol driven procedures. Protocols should be detailed and address:

- Annotations and calculations used in measurements of anatomy or pathology
- Standardized abbreviations, codes, and acronyms
- Standardized scanning techniques allowing for all radiologists to see all examinations in the same scanning order on every patient every time

Most scanning protocols can be preloaded into each scanner allowing the sonographer to push one button for the protocol to populate the scanner. This prepopulated list is used by every sonographer to ensure consistency in imaging. This also allows for reductions in scan time by keeping the focus on the specific exam and reducing the amount of repetitive scanning.

Vascular Access for Imaging Procedures

A large number of procedures require the injection of contrast media to enhance the exam and assist in the diagnostic interpretation. The concern and risk is using the wrong type of line or too small of a gauge of needle that may cause injury to the patient or the inability to complete the exam. Following are some guidelines for developing vascular access protocols:

- Dialysis lines and subcutaneous ports are not to be used for contrast infusion.
- When peripheral IV access is not available, contrast can be injected through a PICC line or other central line if a nurse or physician accesses the line, and it must be labeled "for IV contrast use."
- Power injector limits for PICC lines must be strictly adhered to.
- IV access for pulmonary embolus (PE) studies or CT angiograms (CTAs) should be monitored and updated to the latest technology advancements and best practices.

Listed below are further examples of lines that should not be used for PE, CTA, or other dynamic enhanced scans. These lines either cannot accommodate the injection rates required by these studies or can be damaged by the power injector:

- Any IV in the hand, wrist, or lower extremity
- Any IV smaller than 20 gauge
- Portacath (unless specifically designed to work with power injectors)
- Regular PICC lines
- Any other central line

Patient Safety

In consultation with the medical physicist, facilities should have in place and should adhere to policies and procedures (in accordance with ALARA) to vary examination protocols to take into account patient body habitus, such as height and/or weight, body mass index, or lateral width. The dose reduction devices that are available on imaging equipment should be active or manual techniques should be used to moderate the exposure while maintaining the necessary diagnostic image quality. Periodically, radiation exposures should be measured and patient radiation doses estimated by a medical physicist in accordance with the appropriate ACR Technical Standard.[3]

Various forms of contrast media have been used to improve medical imaging examinations. The value of contrast media has long been recognized as significant, as shown by its common daily utilization in imaging facilities. Like all other pharmaceuticals, however, these agents are not completely devoid of risk; therefore, exam protocols must be established. See Box 4.6 for a sample policy on contrast reaction screening.

Adverse side effects from the administration of contrast media vary from minor physiological disturbances to rare severe, life threatening situations. Protocols for prompt treatment of contrast media reactions must include preparation for the entire spectrum of potential adverse events and prearranged response planning with availability of appropriately trained personnel, equipment, and medications.

Contrast-induced nephrotoxicity (CIN) implies that impairment in renal function (an increase in serum creatinine by more than 25% or 0.5 mg/dL) has occurred within 3 days following the intravascular administration of contrast and the absence of alternative etiology. It is more than likely that CIN that develops after IV contrast injection will have some deleterious effect, particularly on patients who suffer from advanced renal impairment (glomerular filtration rate [GFR] <30 mL/min) before contrast administration.[4]

Gadolinium is widely employed as a contrast agent for MRI and has generally been considered safe. As with iodinated radiocontrast, concern for CIN existed with gadolinium contrast as it possessed many similar qualities (hyperosmolar, renal excretion via glomerular filtration). Early studies in low-risk patients suggested a benign renal profile; however, recent studies raise the possibility of nephrotoxicity. In addition, reports of a previously rare condition entitled nephrogenic systemic

Box 4.6 Sample Policy on Contrast Reaction Screening

ABC HOSPITAL
MEDICAL IMAGING DEPARTMENT

CONTRAST MEDIA DRUG INTERACTION FORM

SCHEDULING FORM

Patient Name: ____________________ DOB: ____________________
Age: ____________________ Sex: ____________________
Weight: ____________________ LMP: ____________________

Accession #: ____________________ Date of exam: ____________________
Type of exam: ____________________ MR #: ____________________

Physician: ____

Diagnosis/Symptoms: ____

Comments: ____

Current Medications: ____

Allergies: ____

Allergic reaction to contrast media? YES/NO Pre-medication given? YES/NO

Type of reaction:
❑ Nausea/Vomiting ❑ Hives ❑ Swelling (where)______________
❑ Trouble breathing ❑ Drop in blood pressure/shock
• Other ____________________

Pharmacist Review

The following medication may increase the risk for renal toxicity:

• Avandamet • Glucophage • Glucovance • Glumetza® • Fortamet® • Metformin

• Metformin/Glipzide • Metformin/Glyburide • Metformin/Rosiglitazone

• Ryomet®

Patient I-Stat/Serum Creatinine:________ Date:_________ eGFR:____________

If the patient is taking any of the above medications, there is a potential allergy conflict; if eGFR is below 60, radiologist must review prior to proceeding with examination.

Pharmacist: ____________________ Date: ____________________

❑ OK to proceed ____________ ❑ Potential allergy conflict

❑ Physician must review prior to proceeding

Physician: ____________________

Fax to Pharmacy ______2689__________ Please fax back to ____________________

fibrosis (NSF) have recently emerged in patients with advanced kidney disease and have been linked to exposure to gadolinium contrast.[5]

Protocols recognizing areas of high risk including contrast media use will assist in directing the facility's focus appropriately. In response to known research and national patient safety concerns, the following steps should be taken, understanding that all policy development and content is organization specific:

- Standardize policy and procedures for administering contrast.
- Standardize forms for prescreening adult and pediatric patients undergoing an IV contrast study.
- Standardize policy for contrast reaction screening.
- Standardize policy for the treatment and reporting of adverse contrast reactions.
- Provide discharge instructions for patients having had an IV contrast study.
- Standardize policy for IV access for exams requiring contrast injections.
- Standardize policy on storage and product recall.
- Standardize policy on contrast extravasations reporting.
- Standardize policy on contrast nephrotoxicity risk screening.
- Standardize policy for gadolinium and NSF.

To maintain a proper understanding of the use of contrast media and potential dangers, a continuing education training program should begin with staff member orientation and include an annual review of both radiology and nonradiology personnel who may come in contact with contrast media usage.

Imaging medications have not historically been handled like other medications within healthcare organizations. In 2004, The Joint Commission mandated that contrast agents and radiopharmaceuticals be treated as medications, subject to the scrutiny of Medication Management (MM) Standards and medication related National Patient Safety Goals (NPSGs). This change ensures that the same controls that exist for other medications within the organization in regards to prescribing, dispensing, storage, security, administration, and monitoring must also be in place for contrast agents and radiopharmaceuticals. Imaging facilities have established protocols on the safe handling of contrast agents and radiopharmaceuticals.

Additionally, an understanding of the role of regulatory agencies in governing the healthcare environment is required of radiologists, radiographers, and imaging administrators to meet the many standards of compliance. Regulatory agencies may be classified into two groups: voluntary (eg, The Joint Commission and Leapfrog) and involuntary (eg, governmental agencies mandating regulatory compliance with local, state, or federal laws—CMS, NRC, FDA, and state licensing laws). Protocols should be put into place outlining continued monitoring and maintenance of all regulation requirements which will ensure compliance at all levels.

Managing Patient Handoffs

In 2006, The Joint Commission instituted NPSG 2E which mandated institutions to "implement a standardized approach to 'hand off' communications, including an opportunity to ask and respond to questions."[6]

Patient handoff is an often overlooked aspect of patient care management in imaging. Outside of interventional procedures, which may require both pre and post observation along with intervention from both nurses and physicians, most imaging staff have a minimal amount of caregiver interaction. However, even if patient interaction is only for a few minutes, during that time the patient's condition may change. How information on the patient's condition is relayed to the next person is critical.

Communication failures are generally considered to be a contributing factor to adverse events in patients. When creating a handoff protocol, some important issues to be considered are:

- Identify handoff situations (eg, transferring complete or temporary responsibility for a patient's care for a period of time, transferring clinical information between healthcare workers).
- Describe essential features of effective handoff communication.
- Recognize barriers to effective communication between care providers.

SIDEBAR 4.1: What Is SBAR?

S—Situation: What is happening at the present time?
B—Background: What are the circumstances leading up to this situation?
A—Assessment: What is the problem?
R—Recommendation: What should be done to correct the problem?

SBAR is a technique for framing conversations about patients that require attention and action. It sets the expectations for the critical information that should be ascertained before contacting the physician and communicated to define the patient's problem and formulating solutions. It ensures that relevant and important pieces of clinical information are communicated every time and sets the expectations of how the critical information should be presented, which is essential for developing teamwork and fostering a culture of patient safety. So no matter the shortness of time spent on an imaging procedure, technologists need to be aware of changes that are taking place with their patients and be able to communicate those changes when necessary to ensure the patient's well being.

- Describe processes already in place that facilitate transfer of information.
- Demonstrate the use of the SBAR technique in communicating patient information (see Sidebar 4.1).

The goal of optimizing handoff of patient care information is to eliminate errors and improve outcomes, which requires the following:

- Pertinent patient historical data
- Information on previous treatment, care, services, reports, and so on
- Information on most recent treatment such as care, services, and reports
- Accurate and up-to-date information
- Communication with limited or no interruptions
- Adequate time allotted for communication
- Interactive communication
- Simple language
- An information verification process

A formal written policy detailing the appropriate steps to be taken during a handoff procedure will decrease the likelihood of adverse events when transferring care between caregivers.

Staff Training

In order to keep pace, an organization needs to consistently update its basic competency requirements by aligning the basic knowledge of staff with the equipment they use every day. Protocols should not be generic in nature and protocol requirements need to be modality specific. Installing an upgrade or putting a new procedure in place constitutes an initial competency. After the initial competency period has ended, it then becomes a basic core competency and should be reviewed annually and incorporated into new technologist orientations.

Review of staff work levels should entail inquiries into dedication to only working on a single piece of equipment, room utilization, and workload distribution (ie, why some staff do all the high-acuity cases and others do nothing but portables). Having an active in-service program using radiologists, staff, and even outside speakers is not only important for technologists to pursue continuing education for licensure but also to maintain a high level of work proficiency. As part of ongoing training and evaluation of work performance, a comprehensive image quality program should be established. This program includes image review and feedback from the reading radiologists and retrospective reviews from the manager or supervisor on how well each technologist is performing. Programs can be designed using PACS/RIS systems, or manually tracking data to monitor quality of procedures and adherence to established protocols.

Evaluate Results: Critical Results Reporting

Although it is expected that a complete, official interpretation will be generated for all examinations and procedures, certain circumstances require results be communicated to the referring physician more quickly than is possible with routine report dictation. As a result of The Joint Commission's NPSG 02.03.01, it is now a requirement that imaging services have a standardized protocol for reporting critical results. The criteria describing what constitutes a critical result are outlined in the ACR Practice Guidelines for Communication of Diagnostic Imaging Findings that went into effect in October 2005.[7]

Even in the absence of a request of a "stat" reading, unexpected or potentially life threatening findings require a summary report or pertinent findings to be conveyed to the referring physician directly. It must also be realized, unlike abnormal laboratory values, the decision to directly communicate findings is fully dependent upon the interpreting radiologist and the history available at the time of examination review.

While The Joint Commission does not specify the maximum amount of time allotted to relay critical results to the ordering physician, it does advise to include time from when the exam is ordered until the result is received. Most imaging facilities strive to achieve 60 minutes or less for critical results reporting. It is also important to track critical results reporting as a quality measure to ensure the standards set forth and agreed upon by the organization are met.

Conclusion

The practice of medicine involves not only the science, but also the art of dealing with prevention, diagnosis, and the treatment of disease. There are many indications for having a radiographic procedure, but there are rules to be followed. There needs to be sufficient clinical indication to warrant the performance of the study and reasonable expectation the results of the study will influence the treatment of the patient. Some specifics to be written into various protocols are:

- The written or electronic request should provide sufficient information to demonstrate the medical necessity of the procedure being ordered.
- Documentation which satisfies necessity includes relevant history and/or a diagnosis if known with appropriate ICD-10 code.
- All images taken are to be labeled with patient identification, organizational identification, examination date and time, the proper marking of the anatomical site, and any other information specific to facility or accreditation requirements
- All imaging facilities should have protocols for standard views, which optimize diagnostic information while minimizing radiation exposure.
- Appropriate collimation and shielding should be used ensuring optimal radiation protection.
- Proper training and adherence to protocols minimizes repeat examinations.

References

1. American College of Radiology. Clarification on PQRI Measure #145 – exposure time reported for procedures using fluoroscopy. Available at: http://www.acr.org/SecondaryMainMenuCategories/quality_safety/p4p/FeaturedCategories/QI-News/PQRIMeasure145.aspx. Accessed January 26, 2010.

2. Beyer T, Antoch G, Müller S, et al. Acquisition protocol considerations for combined PET/CT imaging. *J Nucl Med.* 2004;45(1)(suppl):25S-35S.

3. American College of Radiology. ACR practice guideline for the performance of high-resolution computed tomography (HRCT) of the lungs in adults. Reston, VA: ACR; 2009:3.4

4. Morcos SK. Chronic kidney disease: CT or MRI?: contrast-induced nephrotoxicity. *Appl Radiol.* 2008;37(5):19–24. Available at: http://www.medscape.com/viewarticle/575086_2. Accessed January 26, 2010.

5. Perazella M. Gadolinium-contrast toxicity in patients with kidney disease: nephrotoxicity and nephrogenic systemic fibrosis. *Curr Drug Safety.* 2008;3(1):67–75. Available at: http://www.ingentaconnect.com/content/ben/cds/2008/00000003/00000001/art00010. Accessed January 26, 2010.

6. The Joint Commission. 2006 national patient safety goals. Available at: http://www.jointcommission.org/PatientSafety/NationalPatientSafetyGoals/06_npsgs.htm. Accessed January 26, 2010.

7. American College of Radiology. ACR Practice Guidelines for Communication of Diagnostic Imaging Findings. 2005. Available at: http://www.acr.org/SecondaryMainMenuCategories%2fquality_safety%2fguidelines%2fdx%2fcomm_diag_rad.aspx. Accessed January 26, 2010.

2 Marketing Imaging Services

In this section:

Chapter 5

Review Basic Marketing Principles

J. Lynne Dodson and Luis O. Marquez

Healthcare leaders have come to realize that many marketing principles—long applied in a wide range of manufacturing, retail, and service businesses—have a role to play in the healthcare business as well. These include the core aims of marketing to identify the customers' needs and seek to meet them while bringing value to the enterprise. Marketers accomplish these objectives by carefully analyzing their services, patient base, environment, and competitors; building customer relationships; devising marketing strategies that often focus on product, price, place, and promotion; creating marketing plans that outline goals, objectives, and actions; and finally, implementing those plans and measuring the results.

The application of marketing principles and strategies to healthcare, including to imaging services, is a relatively recent development. The need for a marketing orientation arose with the growth of competition as imaging services expanded from a strictly hospital-based venue to a mix of inpatient and outpatient settings. Technologic developments permitted outpatient imaging, and radiologists soon saw the opportunity to increase revenue by owning radiology equipment, operating freestanding imaging centers, and capturing technical component revenue in addition to compensation for interpreting the images. More recently, competition has expanded to include nonradiology specialists (eg, cardiologists who offer interventional radiology) and nonphysician entrepreneurs.

The proliferation of freestanding imaging centers has resulted in increased market fragmentation. Both hospitals and independent imaging centers have found themselves in competition for patients who previously had little choice in selecting an imaging provider. Marketing introduced not only new business principles, but also an entirely new way of looking at patients, referring physicians, and health plans as customers.

Defining Marketing and Understanding Why It Matters

The focus of the entire field of marketing has also changed over the years, influencing how healthcare marketing is applied. In mid 2004, the American Marketing Association issued an updated definition for marketing[1]:

> "Marketing is an organizational function and a set of processes for creating, communicating and delivering value to customers and for managing customer relationships in ways that benefit the organization and its stakeholders."

A close examination of this definition will help explain what marketing is—and is not. First, the customer must receive value and the organization must benefit. Marketing involves both sides of the same coin—not simply selling a product or service to make money for the organization, but also meeting the customer's needs in a way that he or she perceives as worthwhile. Second, communication is part of the marketing process, but not the entire process. A common misconception is that marketing is about advertising, creating a logo, or getting an article published in the local newspaper. Indeed, these are tactics used in marketing communications, but a great deal must happen before these and other tactics are applied, if at all.

Most importantly, marketing is about customer relationships, not simply transactions. This is especially true for hospital-based imaging departments, which are more dependent on patient referrals than are freestanding imaging centers.[2] Relationship building implies a long-term commitment that must be consistently applied, even if it does not always produce immediate results. Getting such a commitment from senior management may present a challenge. Some of the justifications for applying a marketing focus to a healthcare setting include the following.

Need to build awareness: Although referring physicians (and their scheduling staff) still account for many appointments, healthcare consumers have become much more involved in their own care, including where they receive care. Marketing offers a way for providers to make consumers aware of available services and capabilities.

Need to enhance visibility and image: When multiple providers offer similar services within the same geographic area, marketing is essential to distinguish one from the others and build "top-of-the-mind" awareness.

Need to build market share: Because marketing builds relationships, it can help retain patients (eg, a woman will return each year for her mammogram). When done effectively, it can also bring new patients into the practice, either by attracting them away from other providers or, in growing communities, by attracting them as their initial need for imaging services arises.

Need to influence consumer decision making: By meeting consumer needs and providing information, the marketing process can be a powerful tool to influence a consumer's decisions about undergoing an imaging procedure and selecting a service provider. Marketing efforts targeted to a referring physician's scheduling staff, for example, can lead them to choose one imaging practice over another because it best meets their needs and those of their patient. For screenings such as mammograms, healthcare consumers must first decide that the test is worthwhile before choosing a provider; marketing can influence both decisions in favor of one provider over another.

Need to attract high quality medical staff and employees: With increasing competition for competent staff, most imaging facilities must include prospective employees and physicians in their marketing plans. The marketing process is invaluable to identify the needs of prospective employees, communicate how working for the facility will meet those needs, and bring long-term benefits to both the employee and the organization.

Every staff member is part of the marketing process, from the cleaning staff that ensures the waiting room is spotless to the radiologist who promptly calls the referring physician with a report summary. Effective marketing requires that everyone see the facility from the point of view of the customer (ie, patient, family member, referring physician, community, or insurer) and act accordingly.

Differentiating Healthcare Marketing

Healthcare has a number of unique features that make its marketing challenging and different from that of other industries. First, as a professional service rather than a product, healthcare is intangible and variable. It may be among the most intangible services because its consumers can neither sample before purchase nor effectively evaluate afterwards.[3] Because services cannot be produced and stored for use later, they are considered perishable. In addition, healthcare services are generally consumed simultaneous to production. One marketing challenge that results from these characteristics is the need to balance patient load with available staff and equipment.

The variability of any humanly provided (as opposed to machine-based) service is widely attributed to its subjectivity. In healthcare, efforts to reduce variability in both the types and quality of services have led to such things as evidenced-based medicine and an intense focus on various quality initiatives. Patients may not present with exactly the same symptoms or need for services nor will they respond to treatments in exactly the same manner. Healthcare remains a highly heterogeneous service.

Second, healthcare services and especially imaging services are often highly technical and difficult to describe, especially to lay consumers who are the end users.

In the case of new technologies, even referring physicians may be initially at a loss to understand how the development will improve the patient's outcome or produce other benefits. Even less clearly defined are services such as quality of care or elimination of disease, which are often difficult to measure.

Third, healthcare is a highly personal service with a strong emotional component.[4] This is particularly true of imaging services. Both diagnostic and clinical radiology are often associated with a cancer diagnosis. For the pregnant woman, ultrasound carries the potential to reveal serious problems with her fetus. And in some other modalities there are risks of overexposure to radiation and of the occurrence of iatrogenic morbidity and mortality.

Fourth, patients often use groups of healthcare services during a given episode, especially in the hospital setting. To a patient with cancer, for example, it may be difficult to distinguish between a series of diagnostic radiology examinations and therapeutic radiology procedures. Patients may be unable to discern how a chest x-ray contributed to their outcome or distinguish the radiologic technologist from the radiologist.

Finally, perhaps no feature of healthcare services in the United States has a more profound effect on marketing than the third-party payer system with its gatekeepers and disconnect between end user and payment.[4] Other products and services are subject to laws of supply and demand, and consumers are usually willing and able to negotiate a better price or select another seller. For healthcare services, however, many regions experience a shortage of providers, especially of specialists, leaving patients with few choices. Even in competitive markets, individuals who are covered by managed care plans may find their choices limited by plan gatekeepers. Thus, marketers face a situation in which the end user is often not the decision maker. For patients covered by insurance, cost has historically not been a consideration since the end user and often not even the physician have known the cost of services ordered. Recent efforts to reign in costs through managed care negotiations with providers have attempted to introduce a cost-control mechanism to replace market forces, but the end users remain largely oblivious to the cost of their healthcare. Only individuals who pay out of pocket, either because they are uninsured or because they are undergoing an elective procedure not covered by their insurance, can theoretically be influenced by cost. Yet they will seldom bargain for the lowest price so marketers must find ways to compete on other factors.

These and other qualities have a significant influence on what healthcare marketing does and does not do, can and cannot do. Unlike marketers in other arenas, healthcare marketers usually lack significant industry-wide data on which to base their strategies. Concerns over patient privacy, and the fragmented, local nature of healthcare interfere with the compilation of useful consumer data, including the characteristics of appropriate target markets. So marketers must frequently compile their own, local data before devising their strategies.

Relationship building and other marketing efforts must frequently target the intermediaries (eg, referring physicians, third-party payers) rather than the end users. However, building trust and following a high ethical standard are major points regardless of the user. This is particularly relevant when breaking into new markets. Also, advertising and other traditional tactics may be of little value, for example, in convincing a managed care plan to include a new imaging center on its roster.

Even the fundamental marketing concept of *demand* presents the healthcare marketer with dilemmas. Although everyone will need health services during their lives, a relatively small percentage will need a specific practice's services at any given time, which may make the cost of marketing per patient relatively high. In addition, the demand for many health services is inelastic and likely to arise with little predictability.[4] Except for elective procedures and screening examinations, the need for healthcare services tends to be associated with illness, creating "a disconnect between the service and the anticipated need."[4] Demand for healthcare services is also significantly influenced by accrediting and governmental agencies, which increasingly scrutinize providers for their utilization practices. Societal struggles over the cost of healthcare focus on utilization (ie, demand) as a mechanism to reign in costs, thus artificially controlling demand and countering marketing efforts.

Despite the many differences between healthcare and other services and the impact those differences have on healthcare marketing, the process of marketing strategy and planning remains much the same. Many of the traditional tactics can be adapted and put to good use.

The Four Ps of Marketing

The marketing process involves devising a strategy, creating a plan to achieve the strategy, and then choosing the tactics that will achieve the plan. To create a viable plan, the marketer must make a series of decisions that relate to the target market and to the "Four Ps" of marketing: product, price, place (distribution), and promotion. The unique qualities of healthcare services influence the way in which these four elements are defined and applied by healthcare marketers. The four are interrelated and decisions about one will generally influence decisions about the others.

Product as a Factor in Healthcare Marketing

In addition to clinical services, a number of activities and features should be considered within the scope of *product*. These include the radiologist's report, patient confidence, and customer satisfaction, which can be influenced by everything from staff behavior to the comfort of the examining rooms. Using cutting-edge technology may be a product consideration that will influence referring physicians to send their patients to one imaging facility rather than another, as will the quality of images and the access referring physicians are given to those images.

Radiology practices can build their patient base and increase their revenues by changes in their products that meet their community's needs. Marketers view products in groups, referred to as product (or service) lines. The products within a line are marketed to one general market; they share some characteristics, customers, and/or uses and may also share technologies, distribution channels, or prices. Diagnostic radiology is one example of a product line and a facility can increase its product line "width" (ie, the number of product lines offered) by adding therapeutic radiology services. A merger between an oncology group and a radiology group is another example of increasing product line width. Product line "length" refers to families of products within a line; an example of expanding the diagnostic product line length may be the addition of PET to a facility's service offerings. Finally, adding services to a specific family of products expands the product line "depth," such as when a facility adds pediatric ultrasound to its existing offering of adult ultrasound scans.

As marketing planning gets underway, questions related to product may include:

- What trends could lead to demand for additional services?
- What services currently offered are no longer needed?
- How could existing services be expanded or changed to serve new categories of customers or meet new needs of existing customers?
- Can customer satisfaction be increased and, if so, what changes are needed?
- What is the best way to describe the facility's services to prospective patients? To referring physicians?

Price as a Factor in Healthcare Marketing

In healthcare marketing, price considerations relate not only to the actual price charged for a service, but also to issues such as whether to accept Medicare or Medicaid reimbursement, whether to accept insurance company usual and customary rates, what terms to negotiate with managed care plans, and how to control costs. Traditionally, pricing was not a significant factor in marketing healthcare services in the United States. However, efforts to control what have come to be perceived as out of control healthcare costs through managed care, diagnosis related groups, government intervention, and other means have meant that few facilities can overlook pricing as they develop their marketing mix.

Some marketing strategies will use price as one of the defining features, using tactics to undercut, match, or lead the competition. In healthcare, those who choose to present themselves as the low cost provider must counteract the tendency of people to equate low cost with poor quality. "Few people want to think that they are receiving 'cheap' (poor quality) care."[3] If a facility decides to match its competitors on price, then product, place, and promotion must play a much larger role. Finally, a facility that experiences strong demand for one or more of its services may be able to position itself as the price leader. In doing so, however, it must target customers who are able to pay, accept that it will be unable to serve some patients, and be able to meet customer expectations for service and amenities commensurate with the price.

Among the questions to ask during the planning process related to price are:

- How will prices be determined?
- What prices are being charged for specified services within the geographic region?
- Can revenues from some services cover other services provided at below cost?
- How do practice costs currently relate to pricing? Can costs be reduced without decreasing service levels or quality?

Place as a Factor in Healthcare Marketing

In marketing, issues of place relate to the distribution of the product or service. The most obvious of these considerations are location and office hours. Other elements that are considered "place" issues include parking, patient access, proximity to the target market, waits for appointments, ease with which referring physicians can access reports and images, and office layout.

For purposes of marketing planning, examples of questions related to place include the following:

- Do the current office hours meet patient needs?
- What is the current lag time from calling for an appointment to visiting the office? Should this be shortened? If so, what is the best way to accomplish this?
- Should the facility establish a satellite office? If so, what are the alternatives?

Promotion as a Factor in Healthcare Marketing

Promotion, the most commonly recognized aspect of marketing, encompasses the tactics that will be used to communicate about the imaging facility and its services to the target market(s). Unlike traditional marketing, healthcare marketing tends to have an educational focus that seeks to build relationships rather than sell a product. In other words, healthcare promotion is aimed at getting "the consumer to go to the right place at the right time to receive the right care."[4]

Healthcare marketers have a wide range of communication options, with the choice based primarily on the target market(s) identified, the types of services being marketed, budget, and available expertise. Options range from traditional activities such as newspaper advertising and health fair participation to high tech alternatives such as publishing a blog and linking social media to the organization's Web site.

Among the promotion questions that may be asked during planning are the following:

- How do members of the target market get their health information?
- What traditional media (eg, television, newspapers) reach the geographic region the facility wants to serve?
- How did current patients (or referring physicians) learn about the imaging facility and its services?
- What communication mechanism(s) can best present the service(s) the organization wants to promote?
- What expertise will be needed to carry out the communications plan and who is best suited to provide it?

Levels of Marketing

One of the fundamental activities of anyone involved in marketing is to identify the potential customers to whom marketing efforts should be directed. The broader the customer base, the broader the marketing tactics used. Generally, three levels of focus guide strategy: mass marketing, target marketing, and micromarketing.

Mass marketing refers to efforts to reach a large, general customer base or market. Tactics include advertising nationally in major magazines or on network television or sending direct mail pieces to thousands of households. The diverse nature of the audience means the message must be general, aimed to create awareness in the greatest number of people. Although mass marketing tactics were used by hospitals and other healthcare organizations at one time, few do so at present. A facility such as the Mayo Clinic, which serves patients from throughout the United States and abroad, or pharmaceutical companies that use direct-to-consumer advertising may effectively use mass marketing techniques.

For most healthcare organizations (and other businesses), target marketing most commonly guides strategy and tactics. Market *segments* are identified, groups of potential customers with common characteristics or behavior. Segments that have the greatest potential to build a customer relationship are identified, and the tactics and messages are customized to reach one or more of the high potential segments. Market segments can be defined by myriad variables, including[5]:

- Population density (urban, suburban, rural)
- Sex (male or female)
- Education (some high school, high school graduate, college graduate)
- Income (under $20,000, $21,000–$30,000, $31,000–$40,000, etc.)
- Family life cycle (young single; young married; parent of preschooler; older single; etc)
- User status (nonuser of service, former user, first time user, regular user)
- Loyalty status (no loyalty, light loyalty, strong loyalty, absolute loyalty)

Referring physicians can be categorized by rate of referral: those who represent the top 25% by annual referral volume, the middle 50%, and the bottom 25%; those who have never referred patients; and those who have referred patients in the past.[2]

No matter which customer groups this level of marketing targets, it provides a mechanism to prioritize the use of limited marketing resources and to attract one or more preferred groups.

Finally, micromarketing takes target marketing to an even more precise level, focusing on potential markets with narrowly defined characteristics. For example, a mammography center that would like to grow its patient base could develop a micromarketing strategy targeting young married women aged 31 to 40 years who work in the office buildings within walking distance of the center. Micromarketing can be used in conjunction with other target marketing efforts.

The Marketing Process

An effective marketing process involves four key steps: analysis, strategy, planning, and implementation.

Marketing Analysis

As with any strategic process, careful analysis underlies all subsequent marketing activities. Situational analysis evaluates both external and internal factors. For marketing purposes, the external factors include the following.

Competitors—Most imaging facilities face competition, often quite intense, for patients, preferred provider contracts, and referrals. To devise an effective marketing plan, it must be understood who the competition is, what their strengths and weaknesses are, how and to whom they market, and what their response to marketing efforts is likely to be.

Setting—The environment within which healthcare organizations function continues to challenge even the most carefully laid plans. At the macro level, situational analysis should review pending local and national healthcare legislation, trends in scientific developments that could impact technology or best practices, changes in healthcare financing, and cycles of interest in a given treatment or illness (eg, public interest in breast cancer is high, while that of heart disease in women is building). At the micro level, the analysis should look at issues such as the organization's location and building amenities, the local road and transportation systems serving the market, and the status of the region's major employers (especially those offering health benefits) and whether new ones are expected.

Distribution—How imaging services are distributed in a region can influence marketing strategy and planning. Among the issues to explore are where competitors provide services (eg, in highly populated neighborhoods, multispecialty medical campuses, or freestanding suburban imaging centers), the competitors' organizational structure (eg, hospital based nonprofit, freestanding for profit single specialty, or multispecialty practice), and the use of mobile facilities.

Markets—A careful analysis of current and potential markets will ultimately provide the most valuable data in planning marketing efforts. Among the topics to be analyzed are size and characteristics of current customer groups; identification and characterization of potential new customer groups; estimated rates of growth for both categories; customer distribution patterns; health demographics; demand levels for services; and actual and projected profitability rates for the various market groups.

Marketing related internal factors that are evaluated during a situational analysis include the following.

Current situation—Ideally, past and present activities should be analyzed. In addition to characterizing patients as previously noted, the analysis should attempt to answer questions such as: What marketing efforts have been tried and what were the results? How satisfied are current patients and referring physicians? What professional and business skills are available within the organization? If the marketing effort attracts new patients, can the existing staff and equipment handle the additional workload? What promotional skills (eg, public speaking, writing press releases, or organizing health fairs) are available?

Services—The analysis should include an internal audit of the services currently being provided to patients, referring physicians, and other customers, along with a preliminary assessment of services for unmet needs. Services can be ranked according to one or more criteria, eg, revenue generated, patient satisfaction, or capacity. Service analysis can also assess technological adequacy, including whether current devices are fully meeting patient needs and could meet the needs of an expanding patient base and whether marketing to satisfy unmet needs will require purchasing new equipment.

Finances—Effective marketing is a long term commitment. The analysis should identify the level and source(s) of funding for the marketing effort. Fortunately, there are marketing activities for nearly every budget, some costing almost nothing, others requiring thousands of dollars. A realistic assessment of available funds will help focus plans to avoid spending valuable staff time and other resources on expensive efforts that must ultimately be abandoned for lack of funds.

One of the most useful tools to summarize the results of the situational analysis is the SWOT analysis (see Box 5.1). Widely used in healthcare in planning capital expenditures and other major projects, this tool sorts and prioritizes the strengths, weaknesses, opportunities, and threats for the organization. Strengths represent those elements that give the facility a competitive edge over other providers in the market. Thus, providing high quality images is not a strength, because all imaging facilities are expected to meet that standard. On the other hand, an imaging facility that is the first in its market to offer referring physicians the ability to access their patients' images directly from a database could consider that service a strength for marketing purposes. Weaknesses are factors that interfere with the ability to serve patients and thus to compete effectively. Outdated equipment, inadequate parking, fear of public speaking, or a receptionist who fails to greet patients in a welcoming manner are all potential weaknesses. In marketing planning, weaknesses must be corrected or downplayed. Both strengths and weaknesses arise from internal elements.

Box 5.1 SWOT Analysis for Hypothetical Mammography Practice

	Strengths	Weaknesses
Internal Factors	Digital mammography Off street parking Subspecialty certifications All female physician staff Fully integrated electronic medical record	Declining neighborhood around office Staff working at maximum capacity High staff turnover rate Physicians new to private practice Lack of contract with leading insurer
	Opportunities	**Threats**
External Factors	University branch campus opening Ob-Gyn group practice expanded Practice grandfathered under pending restrictive legislation Approached to merge with Women's Health Service Competitor's conviction for lack of certification	Major employer reducing health benefits Highly competitive market for certified technologists State increasing business tax Competitor's conviction for lack of certification Hospital upgrading mammography services

Opportunities and threats, on the other hand, arise primarily from the external environment. Although usually beyond the control of a practice, opportunities represent factors that can be utilized to increase market share or achieve other marketing goals. The addition of a major new employer to the community, closure of a competitor's practice, or construction of a large assisted living facility nearby all represent opportunities, as do internal activities such as the addition of a new specialist or opening a satellite office. Finally, threats represent factors that may cause underperformance or that interfere with achieving marketing objectives, such as legislation that reduces Medicare reimbursement, a cardiologist who adds interventional radiology to her practice, loss of a major employer, or a lack of qualified technologist applicants.

Marketing strategy and the plans that result from it are designed to take advantage of opportunities to minimize or overcome threats, building on the organization's strengths and working around its weaknesses.

Marketing Strategy

Marketing strategy outlines the long-term objectives the organization seeks to achieve through its marketing goals and tactics. The strategy should be well thought out as it provides a framework for subsequent marketing activities.

SIDEBAR 5.1: Pareto's Principle and Marketing Allocations

Deciding how much to invest in marketing to new versus existing customers is not simple or straightforward. Marketing objectives, the size of an organization's current customer base, and the level of available resources all affect the allocation. However, Pareto's Principle may provide some useful guidelines. Italian economist Vilfredo Pareto concluded that 80% of production came from 20% of producers in most cases. This postulate can help marketers allocate resources:

- Existing customers should be ranked by profits generated, not by sales; marketing efforts should focus on the top 20%. This will on average produce an incremental growth rate of 20% per year.
- Existing products, geographic service areas, and/or target markets should be reviewed for revenue levels and costs allocated to identify the 20% that are generating 80% of profits. To plan marketing of new products, service areas, or target markets, the marketer should focus resources on those that have characteristics similar to the top 20%.

Source: Lemberg P. The vital few profit from the 80/20 rule. Flaunt it at your own risk. Available at: http://www.paullemberg.com/80-20.html. Accessed March 9, 2010.

Numerous strategies are available and there will rarely be just one "right" one (Sidebar 5.1). Rather, the strategy needs to meet the needs of the organization; be one that is compatible with its mission, values, and capabilities; and ideally be creative and achieve staff buy in. Some are based on the product (service)/market mix. A facility seeking to market based on an existing service(s) and existing market could develop a market penetration strategy, that is, one that seeks to attract patients from another facility or convert nonreferring physicians into referral sources. A market development strategy, focused on existing services and new markets, could seek to identify and serve underserved geographic areas. A new service development strategy would aim to market one or more new services into an existing market; the strategy could involve modifying existing services, introducing entirely new services, or creating several levels of quality in a given set of services. The final type of strategy based on the service/market mix is a diversification strategy, which involves both a new service and a new market. This strategy could incorporate merging with a nonradiology specialty or identifying an unserved market and developing services to meet its needs.

Among other strategies are[4]:

- **Dominance strategy:** The leader in a market devises a strategy that will ensure the organization remains the leader based on patient load, revenues, or other predetermined criteria (eg, always being the first to introduce a new device in a given market).

- **Niche strategy:** An organization concentrates on serving a specific portion of the general market, based on geography, demographics, or type of service (eg, a mammography center).
- **Flanking strategy:** Rather than targeting the market leader head on, this strategy aims to achieve its objectives by entering markets not served by the leader, offering secondary services not offered by the leader, or attracting patient groups the leader has ignored.

The four Ps (product, price, place, and promotion) of marketing can also provide a strategic focus. Strategies based on product (service) might seek to gain a competitive edge by favorably comparing one set of services against the competitor's. In some healthcare specialties, a strategy based on price is possible and effective, generally in the case of elective procedures for which the patient pays out of pocket. Given the nature of imaging procedures, pricing strategies are not likely to be very effective, however, as patients and referring physicians have no knowledge of competitors' prices and third-party payers often determine what will be paid (no matter what is charged). Strategies based on place are becoming more common in healthcare,[4] especially among specialties such as imaging that can be provided in outpatient settings. These strategies may seek to provide imaging services in satellite offices or through mobile units. A place-focused strategy may also include objectives related to enhanced patient processing, office amenities, and access. Finally, healthcare organizations often choose to devise a promotion-based strategy, differentiating themselves from the competition through the promotional message and tactics used. An imaging facility seeking to build its pediatric patient base might present a message of reassurance and expertise and market primarily through school-based health fairs and advertisements in local parent magazines.

No matter what focus a strategy has, the document should include the marketing goals, the target market(s), a summary of the current marketing mix (the four Ps), and the SWOT analysis. (Box 5.2.) This document forms the basis for the next step, creating the marketing plan.

Marketing Planning

A formal marketing plan guides the implementation of the strategy, serving as a road map for the entire staff to understand and follow. As such, it must have sufficient detail, yet be flexible to respond to detours that occur over the course of the year. Departures from the plan occur, for example, when a new, unanticipated competitor enters the market, a major contract is lost, or another provider's strategic plan derails the status quo. The investment of time and effort in preparing a formal plan, however, is worthwhile, as it takes the organization through the disciplined

Box 5.2 Sample Market Strategy

Overall Strategic Direction

Alpha Imaging seeks to establish itself as the premier diagnostic imaging facility for children in the community, nearly all of whom have coverage under private or state plans.

Goals

The project aims to

1. Provide enhanced services to children to better meet their imaging needs
2. Increase revenues to counterbalance anticipated lost revenues from recent changes in reimbursement rates
3. Build awareness of Alpha as a caring resource for parents and others who care for children

Target Markets

The primary target market is parents of children ages 5 to 15 years living within a 10 mile radius of Alpha. They seek the best care for their children, and most have some form of health coverage for them. As both parents and children will likely be anxious at the time of seeking services, reassurance and stress reduction will need to be incorporated into services.

Secondary target markets are pediatricians, teachers, day-care workers, and others who regularly interact with school-aged children.

Marketing Mix

Product: The current types of imaging services being offered (eg, ultrasound, x-ray) can meet the needs of pediatric patients. However, changes need to be made in related services, including appointment scheduling, patient preparation, and radiologist participation. Among the possible changes to be discussed are having a radiologist available to meet with parents after the examination and hiring a child life therapist to conduct staff training.

Place: The current reception and patient preparation areas need to be renovated to be more receptive to children. Staff schedules may need to be adjusted to accommodate increased appointments between 3 PM and 6 PM weekdays and new Saturday hours.
Price: No changes are anticipated in pricing, although further analysis will be done seeking reimbursement for radiologist and parent consultation.

Promotion: Promotional efforts will incorporate direct mail, community speaking to parent teacher organizations and other parent groups, and participation in several local health fairs. The Web site will be revamped with a parents' resource center, and the local newspaper will be approached about a column on child safety and health, which may also be adapted as a blog.

SWOT Analysis

Strengths: Equipment was recently updated and can accommodate pediatric patients without adaptation. Most of the radiologists and current staff are parents/grandparents, heightening their sensitivity to children's needs. Facility is located in suburban community with a high pediatric population.

Weaknesses: Reception and patient preparation areas are sterile and designed for adults. Some of the radiologists lack warmth with patients. Building and maintaining the Web site has been difficult and lacking in support; no staff appear eager to take on writing or community relations tasks.

Opportunities: Legislation recently took effect to ensure coverage by a state plan to all uninsured children. A large housing development is now fully occupied, substantially increasing the number of children living within 10 miles of the facility.

Threats: At least one large pediatric practice has approached a rival imaging facility about an alliance.

process of reviewing the marketplace, changes in the customer base, trends, competitive activities, and the successes/deficiencies of past efforts.

An additional benefit to a formal plan lies in controlling expenses. With a plan to refer to, the organization will be less susceptible to a knee-jerk reaction in response to competitive activities or less likely to grab a random good idea such as a special advertising supplement or promotional activity that does not meet the goals of the plan.

The scope of the marketing initiative influences the complexity and duration of the marketing plan. The plan for an imaging facility opening in a new market may cover several years and include sections for each of the four Ps, with secondary plans for specific events such as the grand opening. On the other hand, an established hospital-based imaging department that seeks to increase its referrals may devise a six month plan that focuses on services.

The planning process may also include other activities leading to the final step of implementation. In many cases, key elements will be developed and tested before using them with the entire target market. If one promotional component will be a workshop for referring physicians, for example, the content can be developed and presented to a few physicians who are currently referring patients. Based on their comments, changes can be made, if necessary, before the workshop is offered to the entire group. This development and testing process is also commonly used for promotional literature, especially if many thousands of copies will ultimately be distributed, and advertisements.

Marketing Implementation

With sufficient analysis and planning, the implementation step can be relatively easy and straightforward. A useful tool to translate the marketing plans into workable steps is an implementation matrix.[4] This document details each step that must be taken, the responsible staff person, the resources that are needed, its start date, and its completion date. Accompanying the matrix (or replacing it in the case of short-term, limited marketing projects), a Gantt chart or other computer-based project planning tool allows all members of the marketing team to quickly visualize what must be done and by what date (Figure 5.1).

One of the critical aspects of implementation is timing. The success of many promotional tactics, for example, depends on service and distribution elements being in place; for example, running advertisements to generate new patients will ultimately fail if equipment is outdated or scheduling staff lack good telephone skills. Timing can also be affected by external factors. An economic downturn may create exceptional pricing opportunities for newspaper advertising, for example, leading an imaging facility to move forward its plans to promote a new service.

The implementation step should also incorporate measuring the marketing effort, reporting results, and when needed, making changes to improve those results. Outcome measures such as changes in patient volume, referral patterns for the top 10 referring physicians, and number of people attending community seminars provide data that can be compared with pre-marketing efforts or with future activities. These types of data can be compiled and charted with common software. While outcome measures are most commonly thought of, not all marketing tactics will provide measurable outcomes. In such cases, it may be useful to measure process efficiency. These metrics include tasks completed within the designated timeframe; consistency of message among the various components; and appropriate people carrying out tasks.

Measurement will usually take place before, during, and after a marketing initiative, with results evaluated in terms of the objective(s). Short-term projects may involve establishing baseline measures, logging data during the project lifespan, and then tallying the data to assess the project's success or failure. Longer term projects should include interim assessments so that changes can be made if necessary.

Task	Task Lead	Duration (Days)	Start Date	End Date	1/25	2/1	2/8	2/15	2/22	3/1	3/8	3/15	3/22	3/29	4/5	4/12	4/19	4/26	5/3	5/10	5/17	5/24	5/31	6/7	6/14
Market research	John	61	1/29	3/31																					
Analyze community		61	1/29	3/31																					
Conduct focus group		42	2/4	3/18																					
Identify participants		6	2/4	2/10																					
Develop script		22	2/4	2/26																					
Design evaluation instrument		14	2/17	3/2																					
Analyze demand		30	2/1	3/1																					
Grand Opening	Jane	93	3/15	6/17																					
Plan agenda		5	3/15	3/19																					
Invite guests		47	3/15	5/3																					
Design invitations		27	3/15	4/12																					
Compile guest list		14	3/29	4/12																					
Mail invitations		1	5/3	5/4																					
Track RSVPs		42	5/5	6/16																					
Book photographer		4	3/22	3/26																					
Book caterer		12	3/22	4/2																					
Promote event		75	4/1	6/16																					
Advertise in local media		72	4/1	6/13																					
Add to Web site		18	4/1	4/19																					
Get pricing, etc		8	4/1	4/9																					
Design ad		21	5/3	5/24																					
Write & send press release		14	5/10	5/24																					

Figure 5.1 Gantt Chart to Track Tasks for Two Marketing Projects

The Marketing Plan

In its simplest form, the marketing plan seeks to answer this question: "If this is where we are now—and that is where we want to be—what will it take to get there?"

The plan includes one or more goals of the marketing initiative, as outlined in the strategic plan. The goal is a general statement of what is to be accomplished (eg, to increase Alpha Imaging's market share among women in Smithville or to establish Alpha Imaging as an innovative provider of clinical radiology services). For each goal, one or more objectives are set, having the following characteristics:

- They are clear and concise statements of what is to be accomplished.
- They include a timeframe for achievement.
- They are measurable.
- They are ethical and legal.
- They are appropriate for the target market.
- They can reasonably be expected to achieve the goal without any unintended consequences.

Examples of marketing objectives include:

- Increase CT examination volume by 8% within the next 12 months.
- Achieve overall patient satisfaction scores of 96% within the next 6 months.
- Improve referring physician satisfaction scores by 12% in the first 2 quarters of the year.
- Introduce vertebroplasty procedures, with the goal of completing an average of 8 per month by year end.

A goal can have more than one objective, and a major marketing initiative may incorporate objectives for each of the four Ps of marketing (product, place, price, and promotion) (Box 5.3). However, unless a facility has a dedicated marketing team and significant resources, it is likely that the plan will have to prioritize objectives and/or establish a process for achieving them sequentially, rather than simultaneously. One way to prioritize is to focus on one of the four Ps at a time; another is to start with the objective that is considered most achievable, often referred to as the "low hanging fruit." The early success may encourage the team to tackle more difficult objectives or senior management to assign more resources to subsequent marketing efforts.

Box 5.3 Excerpt from Sample Marketing Plan

Goal 1: Provide enhanced services to children to better meet their imaging needs.

Marketing Objectives

1A. Increase the excellent satisfaction rating from 75% to 85% among parents of patients within the next 12 months.

Marketing Tactics

A1. Conduct parent focus group to clarify issues of dissatisfaction.
A2. Conduct "lunch and learn" staff training on special needs of children.

1B. Shorten time from call for nonemergency appointment to final report from 8 days to 4 days within 4 months.

Marketing Tactics

B1. Increase opportunities for appointments by adding 2 hours 1 evening per week and 3 hours on Saturday mornings.
B2. Have staff radiologist who prepares accurate reports with the shortest turn-around time work with other radiologists to adopt best practice.

1C. Decrease the number of "no shows" or incomplete examinations for pediatric patients to fewer than 1 per week within 6 months.

Marketing Tactics

C1. Develop a Parents' Resource Corner on the Web site and direct parents to the FAQs on what to expect.
C2. Establish system whereby parents are called 24 hours before an appointment and asked for any concerns or questions.
C3. Develop optional program to give children a tour of the facility and in particular a preview of the test they are scheduled to undergo.

Finally, the plan should operationalize the goals and objectives by detailing the actions that must be taken. Key actions should be listed, in sequence if timing matters. They form the skeleton on which the implementation matrix is constructed.

If, for example, the objective is to achieve a 96% overall patient satisfaction score within the next 6 months, just how will that be accomplished? Depending on the results of the analysis stage and the strategy selected, actions that could be taken to achieve the objective include:

1. Implement an employee recognition program that rewards exceptional patient care.
2. Conduct patient focus groups to clarify areas of dissatisfaction.
3. Develop an explanatory brochure to be mailed prior to initiation of new service.
4. Develop a guest services program that speeds check in and eases anxiety.

Involving frontline employees in this phase of the marketing plan may be especially worthwhile. As the ones closest to the patient, they may be able to provide valuable insight into how best to meet their needs. Through their professional associations and local networking, technologists and other staff may have knowledge of marketing activities that have been particularly successful for others. Finally, as frontline staff members are likely to be the ones to carry out many of the plan's actions, involving these employees in the development is likely to increase their commitment and willingness to follow the plan.

Conclusion

Although the healthcare industry was slow to take on the formal processes of marketing, its leaders recognized the value of identifying patients' needs and finding ways to meet them that benefit the organization, which is the core of marketing and compatible with the values of healthcare.

With a strategic plan, marketing plan, and implementation matrix created, those responsible for carrying out the marketing effort can move forward with confidence. Everyone understands what is expected of them, what resources are available, and what the results of their efforts are likely to be. If circumstances change, the group can maintain its momentum while revising the plan quickly if necessary. As objectives are achieved, new ones can be taken on in a continuous marketing cycle.

References

1. American Marketing Association. Dictionary. Available at: http://www.marketingpower.com/_layouts/Dictionary.aspx?dLetter=M. Accessed October 27, 2009.

2. Leepson E. Secrets to effective imaging services marketing. *Radiol Manage.* 2005;27(4):28-30, 32-35.

3. Ginter PM, Swayne LM, Duncan WJ. *Strategic Management of Health Care Organizations.* 3rd ed. Malden, MA: Blackwell Publishers; 1998.

4. Thomas RK. *Health Services Marketing: A Practitioner's Guide.* New York: Springer; 2008.

5. Solomon RJ. *Clinical Practice Management.* Gaithersburg, MD: Aspen Publishers; 1991:271.

Chapter 6

Define and Understand Markets

Rich Egan and Robert Jacoby

Defining the market being served by a given imaging facility is critical to overall operational success. This chapter defines the concept of a market, its dynamics, and the various elements that comprise the healthcare market. This chapter also provides an overview of tools that can be utilized to identify competitors and their services.

As many businesses have learned the hard way, not all products or services succeed. One reason is the failure to fully recognize whether a market exists for the service and, if so, whether it is large enough to generate adequate revenues. Describing, understanding, and predicting markets are critical to ensuring the long-term viability of any business, including both hospital-based imaging departments and freestanding imaging centers.

Review the Fundamentals of Markets

A market is comprised of a group of people meeting a set of criteria. First, the individuals must have unsatisfied needs and/or wants for which they seek a solution. Second, these consumers must be willing to exchange something of value (ie, money, goods, services) for the solution. Third, they must be financially able to make the exchange/purchase, and fourth, they must have the authority to make it.

There is another side to the transaction, of course. The group does not constitute a market for a given business unless and until the business is able to meet the group's need. Thus, patients or referring physicians who seek diagnostic scans with an open MRI device are not a market for an imaging center that only owns a closed MRI device.

In healthcare, this process is usually complicated by the participation of several parties in the exchange between patient and provider. There are up to six roles that take place around an exchange[1]:

- Initiator—the person who first recognizes the unsatisfied need
- Influencer—someone who provides information about how the need might be satisfied
- Decider—the person who chooses the product or service to meet the need
- Buyer—the purchaser of the product or service
- Consumer—the user of the product or service
- Evaluator—someone who provides feedback on the product's ability to satisfy

In many transactions, the same person will play all six roles. In other cases, including healthcare, each role will be carried out by a different person or group. For example, a child with an unexplained pain is taken to the pediatrician (influencer) by a parent (initiator); the doctor (decider) orders an X-ray of the child (consumer), paid for by the parent's health plan (buyer). Both the parent and the health plan evaluate the care. Thus, for most healthcare services—including diagnostic and clinical imaging—identifying and analyzing the markets must take a broad view of those involved in healthcare decision making.

Market Segmentation

Most healthcare providers choose to break the entire market into segments that share common characteristics and unmet needs. Doing so recognizes that few businesses can successfully serve all potential customers and allows the provider to customize services to better meet the needs of the selected markets. On the other hand, market segmentation requires significant research which will likely increase costs, and communicating to multiple target markets may increase promotion costs (Sidebar 6.1).

SIDEBAR 6.1: Setting a Market Research Budget

One of the issues every organization must come to grips with when it decides it needs to conduct market research is how much to budget. Among the techniques commonly used are:

- Setting aside a percentage (0.5% to 5%) of the overall marketing budget
- Setting aside a percentage (0.5% to 1%) of sales dollars
- Basing the budget on needs, that is, determining the number of research projects that will be needed based on the year's goals and assigning a dollar amount to each, preferably in consultation with a research professional
- Setting no budget: as the need for research arises, the administrator must find the funds

Source: Kaden RJ. *Guerrilla Marketing Research*. Philadelphia, PA: Kogan Page; 2006.

For segmentation to work, several criteria must be met. A segment must be:

1. **Identifiable and measurable:** Many characteristics can define a market segment, but not all of them can be accurately identified and measured by research in a cost-effective manner.
2. **Substantial:** Theoretically, two people could constitute a market, but it is unlikely to be one that generates sufficient profit or justifies a specific marketing promotion. To be selected, a market needs to be large enough or have enough purchasing power to generate adequate revenues.
3. **Reachable:** The marketer must be able to communicate with the segment using media, direct mail, the Internet, or other means in a cost-effective manner. It is quite possible to identify a group that shares a common need (eg, older women who have never had a mammogram) but have no way to effectively let the group members know XYZ Imaging Center can meet their needs (eg, these women don't all read a specific publication or visit a particular Web site).
4. **Receptive:** A viable market will have indicated its willingness to use (or at least seriously consider using) the promoted service or product. In healthcare, for example, many patients want affordable care, but few want to give up quality or personal care to achieve it. An imaging facility that promoted itself as the lowest cost provider of "no-frills" care might not find a responsive market.
5. **Stable:** The characteristics and unmet needs of the market overall should remain stable over a relatively long period of time, in order that the marketer's promotional activities will not be outdated or out of sync with the market even before they are carried out. While the "window of opportunity" to reach an individual pregnant woman with ultrasound services is only a few months, the needs of the entire market segment of referring physicians is relatively stable and ongoing.

More than two dozen variables can be used to identify segments, ranging from demographic data such as age to psychographic information such as attitudes. These variables can be grouped in three categories of information, with increasing levels of specificity and difficulty in gathering.[2]

At the most basic level are data related to demographics and geography. With minimal research using government documents, trade association reports, financial reports, and the facility's own patient database, the marketer can locate information on age ranges, gender, income, occupations, and locations that will provide a basis for segmenting the overall market (see Table 6.1). The advantages of using basic variables are the speed and lower cost with which segmentation can be carried out. A couple of examples show how the application of segmenting based on geography or demographics helps identify media best suited to the target audience. If an imaging facility wants to build its Medicare practice, advertising in the local senior services

Table 6.1 Five-Year Population Data, Arranged by Service Area and Age Group, for a Hypothetical Imaging Facility

Service Area	*Age Group*	*2003 Population*	*2008 Population*
Primary	00–17	70,121	71,009
	18–44	91,931	94,634
	45–64	44,428	52,136
	65+	20,332	22,374
Primary Total		226,812	240,153
Secondary	00–17	108,200	115,740
	18–44	117,034	128,561
	45–64	48,941	64,135
	65+	16,366	18,855
Secondary Total		290,541	327,291
GRAND TOTAL		**517,353**	**567,444**

magazines might be an effective tactic. A facility seeking to promote a newly opened suburban satellite office might target commuters to the urban location with billboards or local radio advertising during the peak morning and afternoon drive times.

The next level of research offers enhanced precision and more effective targeting of needs. Mid-level segmentation variables relate to current purchasing habits and the environment in which the customers operate. For an imaging facility, among the data sought are the frequency with which customers use imaging services, types of services used (eg, ultrasound, X-ray), and who currently provides those services (Table 6.2). Also, the customers' awareness of the types of and needs for the various imaging services may give an indication of readiness to utilize those services.

Identifying market segments based on these mid-level variables can be useful in making decisions about new services to offer (or those to eliminate), features and benefits to highlight in marketing communications, and communication tactics to use. For example, an imaging facility may seek to focus its efforts on referring physicians. The segmenting research may show that many primary care physicians in the region are unaware of the benefits and uses for imaging devices recently introduced at the facility. A marketing plan to target these physicians might include making a presentation at the local hospital or medical society; setting up a physicians' information page with case studies on the Web site with a letter announcing its availability; and/or sending a short newsletter to the physicians with case studies, research summaries, and service offerings.

Finally, a third level of research is useful to identify variables related to the healthcare environment that may influence customer decisions, such as cultural

Table 6.2 Mid-Level Market Segmentation: Service Providers

Provider	Service (Inpatient/Outpatient)	Annual Procedure Volume
Facility #1	General Radiography	41,088
	CT	16,293
	Ultrasound	8674
	Mammography	7558
	MRI	5437
Facility #1 Total Procedure Volume		**79,050**
Facility #2	General Radiography	17,520
	Ultrasound	7036
	CT	6130
	MRI	5439
Facility #2 Total Procedure Volume		**36,125**
Facility #3	General Radiography	87,830
	CT	32,618
	Ultrasound	14,981
	Mammography	14,176
	MRI	10,649
	Nuclear	7963
	Interventional/Angiography	6294
	PET	1226
Facility #3 Total Procedure Volume		**175,737**

characteristics, the political environment, and legal and regulatory variables. While some of this information can be located from the same sources as those for basic level variables, additional research will probably be necessary, involving some degree of customer contact, such as surveys. Segmentation based on the highest level of variables will involve significant time, money, and effort, but will pay off with knowledge that may be more detailed than that of competitors. For major marketing efforts involving, for example, a multiyear promotion or marketing of a newly renovated facility, the investment in high-level segmentation will likely pay substantial dividends. Variables are primarily behavioral and psychographic, including what conditions influence a decision; what characteristics the customers exhibit; how the services are used; and what impact a customer's personality, attitudes, and lifestyle have on the decision to pursue an imaging service. In addition, segments can be categorized according to the benefits sought by customers, such as level of service or specific features. Below are four groups based on benefits sought that comprise most healthcare customers[3]:

1. Quality buyers, those that want the best service with no consideration of cost
2. Service buyers, those for whom personal, caring service is paramount
3. Value buyers, those who consider quality at a reasonable cost (as they define it)
4. Economy buyers, those who seek the least expensive option

While basic variables describe primarily characteristics of a segment, these high-level variables reflect actual behavior and attitudes and are therefore more useful in predicting how a group of consumers will behave when offered a chance to seek services. An organization planning to open a women's breast care center, for example, will want to understand elements such as what motivates women to seek mammography and related services and why referring physicians select one provider over another for their patients. Such knowledge can guide the entire marketing mix such as selection of service offerings, the facility's location, staff training, and amenities such as valet parking. Using high-level variables also enables the creation of highly specific communications messages that appeal to the targeted customers.

To access information at this level of specificity, marketers will need to work closely with customers, carrying out focus groups, personal interviews, and other sophisticated research.

Conduct Market Research

Market research can be carried out to learn more about all aspects of the marketing mix, including product (eg, the need for new services), place (eg, location of a satellite office), price (eg, optimal price setting), and promotion (eg, advertising recall). Such research can also provide valuable insight into competition, customer satisfaction, and demand for services. While this section focuses on using market research to acquire data about market segments, the principles and process are similar for other research projects as well.

When market research is well thought out and planned, it provides a solid base on which to make sound decisions. It gives the marketer a good picture of customer behavior, helps identify alternatives, and reduces uncertainty and risk. Research helps ensure marketing resources are used effectively by reaching the right customers with the right message about the right services. Lastly, research provides the basis for convincing senior management of the soundness of marketing plans and the need for committing resources to the marketing effort.

To be effective, market research should be[1]:

1. **Specific:** The research should focus on a specific problem or issue.
2. **Systematic:** It should be well thought out and planned and have a goal.
3. **Objective:** Results should not be biased by the researcher or by the process.
4. **Useful:** The information collected should contribute to marketing planning and decision making and not be unrelated to the goal.
5. **Decision oriented:** Once the research has been collected and analyzed, a decision should result.

As with other types of research, market research should also be valid in that it actually measures what it claims to measure; and market research should be reliable that is, its results are consistent. Otherwise, the results will be suspect and decisions based on them may be erroneous.

Research Tools and Resources

When looking for market segment data, both primary and secondary research may need to be carried out.

Primary research

Primary research entails designing and conducting original research projects that will produce data specific to the marketer's needs. Such research can be carried out by consultants who offer a full range of research services from devising a plan to producing a data analysis report (see Sidebar 6.2). Alternately, management may carry out all the research tasks or hire a consultant who deals with a specific aspect of the project such as designing a survey.

The advantages of primary research include:

- **Specificity:** The research addresses only the issues identified by the marketer.
- **Control:** Management decides everything from the geographic area covered to the research time frame.
- **Spending Efficiency:** Dollars are spent on collecting only needed data, generally resulting in more efficient spending than for secondary research, which will often cull needed data from masses of unnecessary information.
- **Exclusivity:** The research information belongs to the organization for which it was collected, which may provide a competitive advantage.

Despite these advantages, primary research has significant disadvantages, especially for a small imaging facility. First and foremost is the cost, which will generally be much higher than that for secondary research. To devise a research plan, design

SIDEBAR 6.2: Hiring Market Research Professionals

An experienced market research consultant can be an invaluable resource to design and carry out an effective research project. To find one that best meets the organization's needs without breaking the budget, note the following:

- Consult the American Marketing Association, the professional organization for marketers and market researchers; local universities for professors of marketing research; or the local telephone directory under "market research."
- Locate a smaller firm or an individual consultant, who will usually have lower overhead.
- Know who will actually work on the project, not just the salesperson.
- Check credentials, including a review of the researcher's resume and client references.
- Look for a researcher with (1) at least 10 years of experience, (2) experience in healthcare, (3) experience working in research for small and medium sized companies, and (4) skill in working with various research tools.
- Speak with the researcher by telephone initially, and if it goes well, meet with the researcher in person.

Source: Kaden RJ. *Guerrilla Marketing Research*. Philadelphia, PA: Kogan Page; 2006.

a valid survey or other tool, apply the tool, analyze the data, and produce a report is expensive. It is also time consuming, another disadvantage. Finally, the process needed to collect the data sought may simply not be feasible (eg, it may be desirable to interview every person living in a specific community, but unless it is a small town, such a project is probably beyond the budget and ability of an imaging facility to carry out).

Primary research tools include those that produce qualitative data, such as focus groups and observation, and those that produce quantitative data, such as various forms of surveys. Personal interviews can elicit both types of data, depending on the questions asked.

Secondary research

Secondary research relies on data that have already been collected either by the organization or by external sources (Sidebar 6.3). For example, patient records can provide information on geography (zip codes), demographics (age), and usage (referring physicians). Other valuable resources for information at little or no cost include:

- Federal, state, and local government agencies, including census bureaus, agencies on aging, economic development, or education

SIDEBAR 6.3: Some Overlooked Secondary Market Resources

- Competitors' annual reports may provide information on marketing plans, new technology or services recently added, or acquisitions
- Competitors' employment advertisements can reveal plans for new services, facility expansion, and staff expertise
- Health fairs may provide opportunities to observe competitors' marketing efforts, learn about potential alliance partners, and gather information about customer needs and wants
- Employee observations both in the office and in their communities may provide insight into unmet needs, demographic trends, and local healthcare trends
- Customer comments and complaints (informal, not collected during a survey or focus group) may reveal unmet needs, details about competitors, and demographic trends

- AHRA, American Medical Association, and other trade associations
- American Marketing Association
- Nonprofit organizations
- Local chambers of commerce
- University business libraries and research departments
- Newspapers and the Internet
- Publications such as *Medical Economics* and *AARP The Magazine*

It may also be possible to purchase useful reports from market research companies, human resource and other business consultants, and banks and other financial services companies.

Despite its name, secondary research is carried out first by most marketers. Doing so may provide direction for the question to be answered by subsequent primary research; reveal problems to anticipate in carrying out the primary research; or even negate the need for primary research altogether. Secondary research also has the advantages of being relatively fast and easy to carry out, especially with the availability of the Internet, and much less expensive than primary research.

The most obvious disadvantage of secondary research is the lack of specificity that often results when data are used that were collected for another purpose; data may not be presented in the format needed or may be incomplete. In addition, the quality of the underlying research may be questionable or at least difficult to determine; the validity and reliability may not be obvious. Another disadvantage arises when data lack timeliness; the underlying research may have been performed several years earlier, yet the report remains available. The fast pace of change in many healthcare issues means making marketing decisions based on out-of-date information is at best risky. While carrying out secondary research may incur less financial outlays than primary research, it is not necessarily inexpensive. In particular, when reports are purchased from marketing research or consulting firms, the cost may be significant and represent an inefficient use of funds if the amount of useful information is not commensurate with the price. Finally, by its nature, secondary information is not proprietary, but is available to everyone, including competitors.

Research Process

Informal research activities such as reading a newspaper article about pending healthcare legislation or asking a patient whether the staff explained a procedure adequately can provide useful marketing insights. But research designed to support key marketing decisions will usually be most useful when it follows a formal research plan involving six steps. Even marketers who hire research consultants can benefit from understanding the steps, in order to better evaluate the consultant's capabilities and results, provide useful guidance and oversight, and understand cost estimates.

Step 1: Identify the problem

The first step is to identify why the research needs to be carried out: what problem needs to be solved or decision to be made. This focuses the other five steps, reducing wasted time and money spent collecting information that might be nice to know but will not help change the status quo. In general, research will (1) explain why something is happening; (2) predict what may happen in the future if something does or does not change; (3) monitor whether a change is having the desired effect; (4) discover new opportunities; or (5) test a hypothesis.[4] With regard to market segmentation, for example, research might be needed to explain why referrals from certain physicians are declining, discover whether a suburban community's needs would justify a satellite office, or test how several proposed changes would affect the third-party payer mix.

Step 2: Specify information needed

The second step in the research process is to specify what information is sought and whether secondary sources can provide some or all of it. If, for example, the research project is designed to discover whether a suburban community's needs would justify a satellite imaging office, the following questions should be addressed:

- What are the community's demographics and how well do they match current patient demographics?
- Are current providers of diagnostic imaging services meeting the community's needs?

- Who are referral sources from the community and what is their potential impact on patient load?
- What if any effect would the satellite office have on third-party payer contracts?

Some of this information is probably available through secondary sources (eg, community demographics from the chamber of commerce or mayor's office, current patient demographics from the facility's database). As with the example, however, most market research problems will call for primary research as well.

Step 3: Design research plan

The third step involves designing the primary research plan, which identifies the general type of research to be carried out and the best tool(s) to do so. Primary research may be (1) descriptive, in that it seeks to describe the current situation; (2) exploratory, which aims to explain a situation or topic that is not well understood by the marketer; or (3) causal, seeking to reveal a cause and effect relationship between variables. Descriptive research works best when demographic and geographic data are sought and is most often used when the research objective is to explain, monitor, or test hypotheses. Exploratory research tends to be less formal than the other types and is used primarily when discovery is the research objective. Finally, causal research is a highly structured design that tests whether changes in an independent variable have an effect on a dependent variable. This research type is used primarily when the objective is to predict or test hypotheses.

As described earlier, the research tools include observation, focus groups, personal interviews, and various types of surveys.

Step 4: Develop and administer tools

The fourth step calls for developing and administering the actual tool(s) to collect the data. In the case of observations, for example, a checklist of actions or behaviors to observe and a scale for noting them may need to be devised. Questionnaires will need to be created for focus groups, interviews, and surveys (see Sidebar 6.4).

In most cases, it is not feasible to use the tool with the entire market, so it will be necessary to devise a means of accurately sampling a representative portion of the population. Among the procedures that can be used are two types of *probability* sampling that allow the extent of randomness to be calculated: simple, in which a group of individuals is selected by chance from the entire market population; and stratified, in which the entire population is categorized into subgroups from which

SIDEBAR 6.4: Seven Questions to Ask Before Administering a Survey

1. Will the survey appeal to respondents? It should be as short as possible, easy to complete, and relevant.
2. Does each question deal with only one concept?
3. Does the scale allow respondents to make a full range of answers? For numerical scales, offering only four options will usually prohibit a neutral answer, which may be desirable from the researcher's point of view but not necessarily from the participant's. Also, when possible include "Other" and room for a write-in answer.
4. Are all questions clear and as neutral as possible? Asking leading questions is a waste of time (eg, "Do you agree that the staff are competent? ❒ Yes ❒ No).
5. Are all questions relevant? Only questions that will actually guide decisions or actions should be included.
6. Would some questions be better answered with observation? If so, they should be eliminated from the survey and an observational study devised to get the necessary answers. This is especially true for customer behavior issues.
7. Does the questionnaire include a mechanism for respondents to provide information that may be unexpected, surprising, or otherwise previously unknown? Providing space for additional comments and asking open-ended questions that require more than "Yes" or "No" answers are among the ways to accomplish this (eg, "If you managed our reception area, what would you do differently?")

Source: Hiam A. *Marketing for Dummies*. Chicago, IL: IDG Books Worldwide; 1997:101-105.

samples are selected at random. Another type of sampling is termed *nonprobability*, in which the sample is selected based not on statistical probability but on criteria such as quotas, judgment of one or more reasons thought to produce a representative sample, or simply convenience (eg, asking for volunteers).

Step 5: Analyze data

The fifth step in carrying out market research is to process and evaluate the data. Raw data should be reviewed for incomplete or inconsistent responses and data entry errors, and they should be corrected or adjusted, as appropriate, without affecting the sampling. The data can then be analyzed using any of several techniques. Simple descriptive analysis of quantitative research, for example, uses charts, figures, and measures of central tendency (eg, mean, mode, median) to describe the results. An example of a chart is shown in Figure 6.1. The results of qualitative research, such as focus groups, may simply be grouped into categories or coded for use in the final narrative report. Using statistical software, the marketer can also evaluate the data using inferential analysis. This technique allows inferences to be made about differences in the data between groups such as whether the differences are the result of chance or are attributable to a specific cause. When research is conducted to devise market segments, inferential analysis can help establish which have the greatest within-segment homogeneity (ie, members

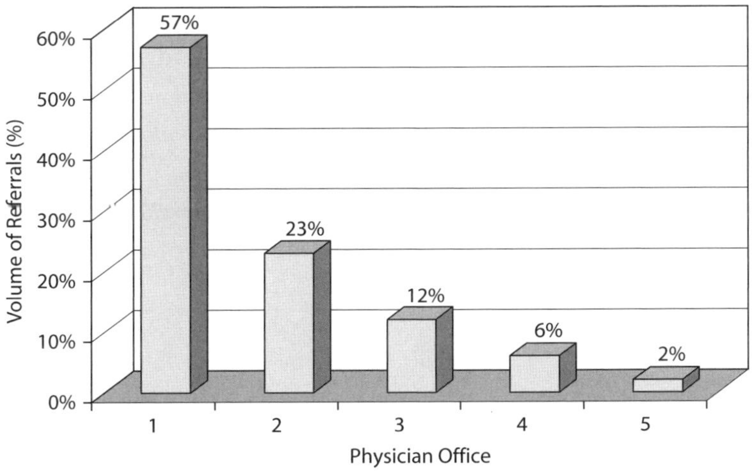

Figure 6.1 Simple descriptive analysis of quantitative research.

have the same characteristics) and which have the greatest between-segment heterogeneity (ie, segments with the fewest similarities).

The question that must be constantly asked when analyzing data is: "Compared to what?"[5] In other words, if survey results show 25% of residents would prefer to visit a satellite office for diagnostic testing, it cannot be known from the isolated data whether this is a satisfactory response. Among the possible comparisons are[5]:

1. **Compare with a control:** This is probably the most common comparison made. The control selected should be one that reflects success, so that meeting or exceeding it guarantees a positive outcome. One example is a survey that asks consumers to choose between A and B, where A is an established market leader or existing successful service and B is the imaging facility being evaluated or a new service. Controls can also be rating goals set by management.
2. **Compare with previous research:** Organizations that repeat research on a regular basis have a distinct advantage in that they can compare each set of new results with the previous ones to establish trends, identify changes in their market segments, and be better able to gauge whether planned changes or new services will succeed.
3. **Compare with industry norms:** Research firms and professional associations will often provide normative data that allows a marketer to compare research results with aggregated data of similar organizations.
4. **Compare with actual behavior:** Certain studies may use data on behavior of existing customers as a point of comparison with the studied group. For example, if an imaging facility wants to increase referrals from several physician groups, it

can choose a control from among the other physician groups that refer patients at the preferred rate. By measuring and comparing attitudes of the two segments, changes that can affect referral rates can be identified.

5. **Compare with alternatives:** If other controls are not available, it may be possible to devise two or more alternatives to be researched and their results compared. Such comparisons are commonly used to evaluate advertising themes, for example; a focus group is asked to respond to several different advertisements for the same service or organization.

Step 6: Prepare a report

The final step in the research process will generally require some form of report, which is discussed at the end of this chapter. The report should enable decisions to be made (even if that decision is to continue the status quo) and actions to be taken.

Profile Market Segments and Select Target Markets

Once the primary and secondary research has been carried out, a profile of each of the market segments in the service area can be created, which can be incorporated into the market report. The profile describes the various segments based on research results that reveal the geographic, demographic, behavioral, and psychographic characteristics, as discussed earlier. The variables chosen should relate to the customers' actual buying habits. The profile will usually also include a summary of each segment's media usage habits, which will help guide marketing communication efforts.

Once segments have been characterized, one or more can be selected that will be the focus of marketing efforts. The selected segments become the target markets, and a marketing plan can be designed to reach them.

In evaluating segments for their potential as target markets, the following key questions should be considered:

1. Is the segment large enough to achieve the marketing objectives?
2. Does the segment show signs of growth?
3. Does the segment meet the practice mission?
4. Is the segment likely to respond to the marketing effort with the desired behavior (eg, refer patients)?
5. Can the practice meet the needs of the segment (ie, does the organization have the skills, knowledge, and expertise to serve these customers)?

Project Market Demand for Services

Before a marketing plan can be designed, another key piece of information that needs to be assessed is the level of demand for its services, especially within the target market(s).

Demand assessment usually begins with the industry overall, then moves to regional and local trends, ending at the facility's own patient database and market research. During the first 5 years of the twenty-first century, the popularity of freestanding imaging centers increased approximately 73%.[6] In all likelihood, hospital-based imaging services will continue to face competition from freestanding centers, as overall demand for imaging services continues to be strong. Several factors contribute to the projected increases in demand, including technological developments in high-end modalities such as CT, MRI, and PET/CT; advances in other medical technologies that depend on imaging (eg, cardiac catheterization); and perhaps most importantly, the lengthening of expected life span of the patient population.[7] Box 6.1 provides a summary of some of the key drivers for increased use of imaging services. Understanding the drivers that will impact the growth, utilization, and demand for imaging services is essential to the development of ongoing operational strategies to meet the increased demand within a given target market.

Because utilization and demand are different for each modality and service, focus should be placed on the services for which the marketing plan is being created. For example, between 2006 and 2016, CT utilization overall is expected to increase between 15% and 60%, MRI between 13% and 50%, and PET and PET/CT from 13% to 120%.[8,9] Yet a review of a facility's utilization data finds that CT utilization has dropped an average of 3% for the past 3 years. Simple trend analysis assumes the trend will continue in a straight line, thus projecting declining demand

Box 6.1 Drivers of Increased Use of Imaging Services

Population (eg, growth, aging)
Disease demographics (eg, increased prevalence of chronic conditions)
New standards of care
New treatments and procedures
Consumerism (eg, increased demand for less invasive procedures)
Emergence of new technologies and applications
Outpatient imaging (eg, expansion of ambulatory services)
Reimbursement policies (note: could also decrease imaging volume)

Source: Sg2. The Edge Report: New Directions in Medical Imaging. 2005; 2–8.

for the next few years. However, demand is rarely that straightforward, so the process should also use research results to identify factors that are likely to affect the demand, in this case for CT services. If older patients use more CT services than younger patients, for example, and young adults have been identified as a target market, the demand for CT tests is likely to continue declining—unless new applications for CT, loss of a local competitor, or another factor intervenes. The likelihood of these various factors occurring needs to be assessed and their potential impact included in the demand analysis.

For larger organizations or hospital-based imaging departments, a technique known as the "jury of executive opinion" might be useful. Each department or service unit manager is asked to project demand within his or her area and for the organization overall. Then estimates are reviewed until a consensus is reached. This technique is popular because it is simple and can be accomplished relatively quickly. It takes advantage of internal expertise, experience, and knowledge of a specific area, rather than requiring one person to delve into all areas at once. It heavily relies on historical data, however, which in a rapidly changing industry such as healthcare may produce faulty forecasts.

These types of analysis are qualitative, but quantitative methods can be used as well. Computer software, for example, makes carrying out sophisticated statistical modeling, such as regression analysis, possible. This technique devises a model incorporating the variables that are likely to affect an event, in this case future demand. Based on research data, the relevant numbers are plugged in and the model forecasts the result. Of course, this technique assumes that the variables that affect demand for imaging services locally are understood and can be quantified.

Another means to project demand is to conduct a market test, in which a new service is introduced to a few specific markets that are representative of the entire set of target markets for the new service. Results from the test can then be projected over the full set.

For more about assessing the operating environment, see AHRA's book *Asset Management in Radiology.*

Analyze the Competition

Within any given market in which goods or services are provided, competition is both inevitable and necessary (Sidebar 6.5). Imaging services are certainly no exception. Because outpatient imaging services have historically been such lucrative

> **SIDEBAR 6.5: "Co-opetition"**
>
> "Co-opetition" is a buzzword coined to describe cooperative competition, which focuses on cooperation between companies in imperfectly competitive markets. For example, a facility with a traditional MRI has a patient who is claustrophobic. It refers the patient to a nearby facility that has an open MRI. Although this facility is in direct competition, it is considered a complementary customer, just one of many types of internal and external customers that all must be dealt with effectively to achieve and sustain success.

sources of revenue, for-profit entrepreneurs have focused their efforts in recent years on meeting outpatient imaging demand, in direct competition with hospital-based services.[10] In addition, "because of fundamental changes within the [healthcare] industry brought about by the influences of managed care, efforts to reduce costs and increase efficiency, and the increasing presence of for-profit healthcare organizations, every segment of the industry has become highly competitive."[11]

Thus, a market study needs to include a competitor analysis, which will help the organization understand local competitive forces, identify competitor vulnerabilities, anticipate competitor actions that could negatively affect an organization's market share, and assess competitors' response to the organization's marketing actions. "Misjudging or underestimating competitors' resources, capabilities, or competencies is a serious misstep."[11]

A competitor analysis includes:

1. **Current competitor profile:** This section describes each competitor according to the services offered, technology, market share, financial strength, target markets, key partnerships and alliances, and recent news items. Wherever possible, it should also include the competitor's report turnaround time, backlog for patient appointments, and key payer contracts in place. A summary of recent marketing activities may also be useful.
2. **SWOT analysis:** Each competitor's strengths, weaknesses, opportunities, and threats should be identified and organized (see Box 6.2). Another tool to assess strengths and weaknesses requires managers to rate his or her own facility and each competitor on key factors (see Table 6.3).
3. **Potential competitor analysis:** Some of the strongest competition may come from the least expected sources—new entrants into a market segment or service area. Cardiologists or oncologists, for example, may add imaging capability to their interventional services. It is also possible that even non–healthcare-related businesses may become competitors: assisted living organizations have found themselves competing with hotel operators, who transferred their guest services

Box 6.2 Sample Competitor SWOT Analysis

Strengths	Weaknesses
■ Local pride, heritage, sense of community ownership ■ Strong reputation across a broad spectrum of services ■ Perception for friendly, more personal caring ■ Widespread recognition for convenient location ■ Physical appearance of the facilities and campus ■ Commitment to investment in new facilities and technologies	■ Emergency department issues have negatively influenced general perception ■ Prevailing perception that metropolitan hospitals to north and south offer superior capabilities, technology, and staff specialists ■ Lack of brand strength compared to heavily marketed big city–based institution
Opportunities	**Threats**
■ Fortify home base by intensifying consumer and physician loyalty ■ Increase referrals and consumer preference in secondary marketing areas ■ Strengthen perception as a community leader by providing information and education ■ Increase recognition of major product line strengths to establish image ■ Use convenience and location to win the day where all things are equal	■ Decrease in volumes in most profitable procedures caused by increased siphoning of business by specialty facilities such as diagnostic imaging centers ■ Loss of volume in other service areas due to: ○ Construction of satellite facilities by heavily marketed organizations to the north ○ Increased expansion of secondary market facilities to the east

knowledge to that of caring for elderly patients. Might a spa add mammography and ultrasound to its business model?

4. **Decision time line:** For key competitors, it may be useful to construct a time line of past strategic decisions (eg, acquisitions, service changes, satellite offices), with an indication of scope and/or size of the activity. A review of the time line can reveal the competitor's strategic direction, which could lead to forecasts of future actions. For example, an imaging practice that has acquired or merged with three other practices over the past 8 years has a strategy of horizontal, external growth. It can be expected to make another acquisition within the next 12 to 18 months, which could have an impact on the evaluating organization's plans to target certain patients currently being served by the competitor.

Table 6.3 Assessment of Strengths for Hypothetical Imaging Facility and Its Primary Competitors

Success Factor	*Facility*	*Competitor 1*	*Competitor 2*	*Competitor 3*
Location	7	9	5	5
Report turnaround	9	9	7	8
Relations with key referral groups	7	6	5	8
Management skills	7	3	7	?
Staff competence	9	9	7	6
Effective marketing	4	9	4	6
Mean	**7.2**	**7.5**	**5.8**	**6.6**

Rating scale: 10 = strongest; 1 = weakest; ? = insufficient information available

Source: Adapted from Solomon RJ. Clinical Practice Management. Gaithersburg, MD: Aspen Publishers; 1991:408.

To compile the competitor analysis, the following questions should be asked:

- What are the unique selling propositions of the competitors? For example, do they offer cardiac services or more specific cardiac CT?
- What marketing strategies do they pursue? Who are their target markets? Do they serve specific niches?
- What are the competitors' customer service capabilities? Do they offer valet parking or weekend appointments, for example? How extensive are their service offerings?
- What are the weaknesses in the competitors' business operations? What are their turnaround times for radiology reports? Do nonemergency patients have a long wait for appointments?
- What is the financial position of the main competitors? Can their profit margin be estimated? More importantly, can they afford the most advanced equipment available in their capital budget?
- What is the quality of the competitors' services? Do they have a positive image within the community at large as well as with their healthcare colleagues?
- How do patients perceive the competitors in comparison with the organization?
- What is the competitors' vision of the future of healthcare and of this community?

A number of primary and secondary sources should be analyzed to answer questions such as these and prepare a useful competitor analysis. Among those sources are local newspaper articles and television news reports; the competitors' marketing materials, annual reports, and Web site; sales representatives and other vendors serving the competitors; their recruitment advertisements; former employees and patients; and healthcare colleagues in the local community. For major marketing projects, it may be worthwhile to conduct focus groups or patient surveys. Having staff members call competitors' offices can provide insight into appointment backlogs, service capabilities, and staff friendliness and knowledge.

To avoid becoming paralyzed by an abundance of competitor information, focus should be placed on the target market(s) or service areas under consideration for the current marketing effort.

Prepare the Market Study

Having collected primary and secondary research data on not only the imaging practice, but also its competitors and the healthcare environment, the findings need to be presented in a format that decision makers will find useful. The size and scope of the research project will usually define the size and complexity of the report. In most cases, the following elements are the minimum that should be included:

1. **Title page**—includes the study subject, for whom the report is prepared, who prepared it, and when
2. **Table of contents**—reports longer than about 12 pages benefit from a table of contents, including a list of figures and tables
3. **Study objectives**—an introduction that provides the general purpose and specific objectives, a statement of limitations, and a brief description of research methodologies
4. **Management summary**—a 2–4 page summary of the key findings in an easy-to-read format (eg, bulleted list)
5. **Conclusions and recommendations**—a short section presenting the researcher's conclusions based on the facts presented and his or her recommendations for action; the researcher's unique perspective can make this section invaluable to decision makers
6. **Endnotes**—numbered text citations should be used for quoted material and full references should be given; if a glossary of key terms is provided (rather than being defined at first mention), it can also be included in this section
7. **Detailed findings**—usually the longest section, it ideally is organized logically (eg, major topics related to each research objective) and includes supporting charts and graphs presenting research data; for focus groups, this section contains more narrative, with quotes from participants and findings that reflect the behaviors and attitudes revealed by each question
8. **Appendix**—may include oversize supporting tables and charts, copies of questionnaires, participant demographics, computer printouts of survey data or statistical analysis, and copies of secondary resources
9. **Storage files**—a CD or other storage device containing all documents used

Ideally, when the report is finished, it is sufficiently organized and complete that someone unfamiliar with the project could understand the report even months after its preparation.

Conclusion

It is imperative to take full advantage of the many primary and secondary sources that currently exist for market data. Organizations that identify their target markets, design their services to meet the markets' needs, communicate effectively to the targets, and understand competitors' capabilities and strategic plans have a strong competitive advantage in what has become a challenging environment in which to succeed.

References

1. Schewe CD, Hiam AW. *The Portable MBA in Marketing*. 2nd ed. New York, NY: John Wiley & Sons; 1998.
2. Target markets and market segmentation. KnowThis.com Web site. Available at: http://www.knowthis.com/principles-of-marketing-tutorials/targeting-markets/market-segmentation/. Accessed November 18, 2009.
3. Kotler P, Clarke R. *Marketing for Health Care Organizations*. Englewood Cliffs, NJ: Prentice-Hall; 1987:244.
4. Planning for marketing research. KnowThis.com Web site. Available at: http://www.knowthis.com/principles-of-marketing-tutorials/planning-for-marketing-research/. Accessed November 18, 2009.
5. Kaden RJ. *Guerrilla Marketing Research*. Philadelphia, PA: Kogan Page; 2006.
6. Business IQ. *Illuminations 2005: Market Trends for Diagnostic Imaging*. Berlex; 2005.
7. Sg2. The Edge Report: new directions in medical imaging. 2005; 2–8.
8. Innovations Center. *Radiology—Future of Diagnostic Imaging*. Innovations Center Business Brief. Washington, DC: Healthcare Advisory Board; 2008:3.
9. Sg2. The Edge Report: smart growth. Presented at: the Sg2 Annual Meeting; July 19, 2006; Chicago, IL;26.
10. Groneman RW. Hospitals scramble to fill shortage of medical technicians. *The Business Review*. June 18, 2004. Available at: http://albany.bizjournals.com/albany/stories/2004/06/21/story3.html. Accessed January 27, 2010.
11. Ginter PM, Swayne LM, Duncan WJ. *Strategic Management of Health Care Organizations*. 3rd ed. Malden, MA: Blackwell Publishers; 1998:95, 103

Chapter 7

Develop a Marketing Program

J. Lynne Dodson and Philip Ruth

An imaging facility that positions itself within its marketplace and builds a strong brand identity has paved the way for an effective marketing program. Once human and financial resources have been identified, a choice from a variety of promotional options must be made, ranging from the traditional tactics of advertising, public relations, and educational marketing and community outreach, to the more cutting-edge tactics of Internet-based media, service line marketing, and social marketing.

Large hospitals and healthcare systems may have marketing staff whose responsibilities include developing and implementing a marketing program for imaging and other services. In most cases, those marketers will rely heavily on the imaging department for data and insight into many elements of the marketing initiative, including positioning, service line characteristics, resources, and the most appropriate tactics for the imaging target markets. Smaller freestanding imaging centers and hospitals may face even greater demands, as they may find themselves responsible for designing and managing the entire marketing program. Either way, they must understand positioning, marketing tactics, and related program elements.

In a geographic area dominated by one hospital or a single imaging center, marketing may primarily be designed to reinforce consumer behavior and intimidate competitors from entering. Even a long-stable marketplace cannot be taken for granted, however. The development of teleradiology, for example, has eliminated traditional geographic barriers to market entry. Complacency and lax service standards among the competition are also opportunities for an aggressive competitor to successfully disrupt a formerly stable situation. Among the key elements that should be in place before a marketing program is undertaken are a clear positioning strategy for the organization and the intelligible delineation of its brand(s).

Position the Organization and Its Brand

In devising a positioning strategy, marketers seek to differentiate their organizations from their competition in the minds of consumers. More than image, a market position also incorporates the consumer's perception and is generally viewed in relation to the competition either explicitly or implicitly. For example, an imaging center that offers only MRI might position itself as the region's only focused MRI provider with expertise developed through thousands of examinations, the implication being that this is preferable to the scattered focus of the competitor's general imaging practice.

"Positioning involves (1) creating a real differentiation and (2) making it known to others."[1] It is crucial, however, that the differentiation be one that represents reality, can be delivered by the organization, and is important to the target audience. "Positioning will not be effective if the target group does not perceive it as meaningfully different.... [T]*heir perception is truth*."[2]

Market positions can be based on a variety of themes. One suggests building on current strengths, as in the previous example of the focused MRI provider. Another premise identifies a target audience that is not currently being well served and focuses on that niche. A third approach attempts to reposition the competition as less than desirable in some fashion.

Overall, a choice of tactic falls into one of four basic positional categories[1]:

Market leader: In mature markets, one organization may assume the leadership position by having an excellent reputation, being the first to introduce new technology, taking part in key clinical trials, organizing opinion leaders regarding legislative issues, and so forth. To maintain its leadership, the organization must have substantial resources to fend off challengers, a commitment to constantly seek to improve quality, and a highly effective distribution system (eg, satellite offices). Strategies need to be developed to protect current market share while trying to expand both total consumer demand and the leader's market share.

Market challenger: An organization may seek to challenge the market leader, another second-tier competitor, or a much smaller competitor. A challenge has better chances of success if the competitor is not currently serving its market well or has insufficient capital to invest in necessary new technology. Challenger strategies include expanding service lines, improving services, introducing innovative services, reducing operating costs (and thereby offering lower prices and/or realizing increased profitability), or enlarging distribution (eg, by acquiring a smaller competitor).

Market follower: Unlike challengers who are likely to stimulate retaliation, followers devise strategies that allow them to grow without using resources to combat a fearful competitor. These strategies, however, do not permit passivity or total "me too" copycats. Followers must retain current customers, maintain consistently high quality while controlling costs, and be open to moving into new markets as they arise. Strategies may focus on (1) following the leader in most markets and service offerings; (2) following in major innovations and distribution channels only, while generally going its own way; or (3) following closely in a few areas and avoiding any direct competition in others.

Market nicher: Position strategies that develop a market niche theme involve finding areas of market specialization that can be profitable yet are of little or no interest to major competitors. Specialization may revolve around the customer, the product, the market, or the market mix. The niche needs growth potential and the organization must have the necessary services and skills to serve the niche well. To avoid the pitfalls of a disappearing niche or a significant competitive challenge, organizations that adopt the market nicher position will generally identify more than one niche for their strategy.

Positioning Via Mapping

An effective positioning statement may have fewer than 10 words. Creating a concise, focused statement takes effort, but that effort will be worthwhile. The positioning statement provides a solid base on which to build all marketing communications. Having a position makes it easier to select tactics and create messages: only those that reinforce the position in the minds of the target audience(s) need be considered, allowing marketing communications to be inherently consistent, which is essential. Also, "by conveying a common positioning, each vehicle of communication will reinforce the others for a cumulative effect, maximizing the return of your marketing investment."[2]

The various techniques to devise a positioning statement require market research on the organization's products/services, the competitors, and the target audience(s). Differences in the techniques arise primarily from the focus, whether it is on product characteristics, competitors' weaknesses, or consumer motivation. One technique uses mapping methodology (see Figure 7.1) to rank the organization and its competitors based on product attributes[2]:

1. The attributes that the target audience considers important are listed on the right side of the chart in descending order of importance on a scale of 10 to 0 shown on the left side of the grid, with 10 being most important.

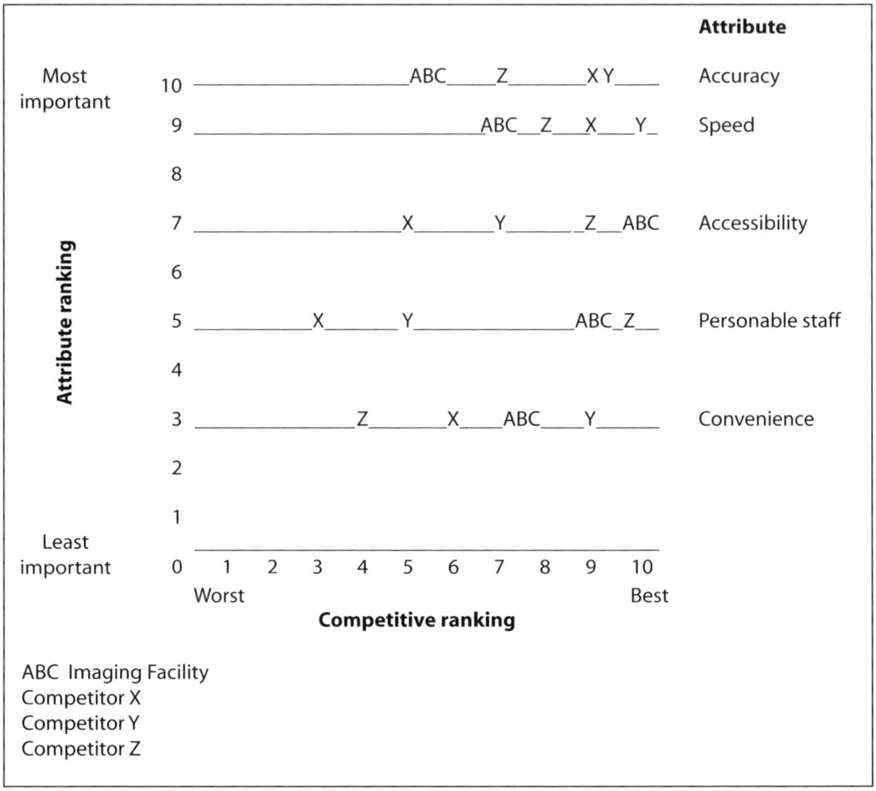

Figure 7.1 Position Map

Source: Adapted from Hiebing RG Jr, Cooper SW. *The One-Day Marketing Plan*. 2nd ed. Lincolnwood, IL: NTC Business Books; 1999:150.

2. For each attribute, the organization and its competitors are each plotted on a scale of 0 (worst) to 10 (best) from left to right, reflecting how well that attribute is currently being served.

3. By examining the organization's ranking on the most important attributes in light of its capabilities and in comparison to the competition, the marketer can begin to identify several possible positions.

For example, ABC Imaging Facility plans to focus its marketing efforts on referring physicians. It has conducted market research, including focus groups and a survey of all potential physician groups in its region. Based on its findings, a position map is compiled (shown in Figure 7.1). On the two leading attributes in importance—accuracy and speed—ABC ranks below some of its competitors, and ranks highest for accessibility. In devising its position, ABC could choose to remain a market follower in these categories and reinforce its position as the accessible provider. On the other hand, if ABC has the resources, capabilities, and willingness to revise its systems to ensure consistent accuracy and high-speed reporting, then it may choose to challenge the leaders with a position statement (and subsequent marketing campaign) that focuses on those attributes.

If research is not available or has failed to provide sufficient data to perform such an analysis, a group of individuals knowledgeable about the organization, its competitors, and the target audience could be convened. Each person is asked to list the most important attributes and rank them from lowest to highest importance; by averaging these, a rank ordering is created. Then by consensus the group identifies the relevant competitors. Again, each member ranks the competitors on each attribute and these are averaged before they are added to the map. Although this approach is not as accurate as one based on primary research, it may result in a more objective map than one created without any research.

Branding

"Branding is the process of establishing and managing the images, perceptions, and associations that the consumer applies to your product, based on the values and beliefs associated with your product."[2] Effective branding is closely associated with an organization's positioning strategy, as both relate to the consumer's image of the organization and each should reinforce the other. The ultimate goal of branding is to build and maintain brand loyalty, that is, to have consumers consistently purchase the brand's services/products to meet their needs. Thus, as one marketing expert has noted, "The art of marketing is largely the art of brand building."[3]

Branding touches every aspect of the organization and is comprised of the entire image that the organization creates with its services and products, including emotional, visual, tactile, experimental, and cultural elements. The branding of a product, service, or organization identifies it to consumers and draws customer loyalty and referrals. Strategically effective and consistent branding will increase:

- Awareness
- Product or service differentiation
- Perceived quality
- Exposure of the brand, symbol, logo, and/or slogan
- Positive associations

Valuable brands have equity beyond that of the products or services they represent. This equity can be represented as a pyramid (see Figure 7.2). Organizations at the bottom of the pyramid must spend considerable marketing resources on promoting their brand, differentiating themselves from their competitors, and finding

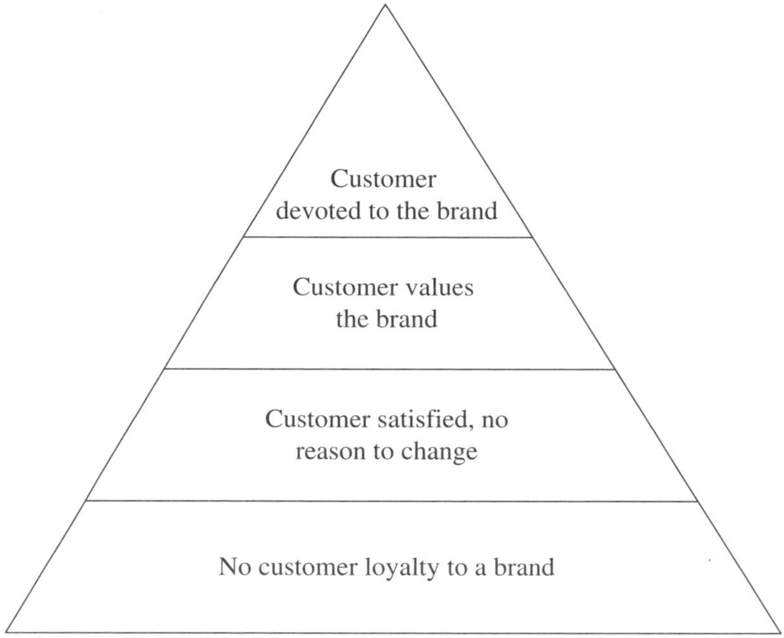
Customer
devoted to the brand
Customer values
the brand
Customer satisfied, no
reason to change
No customer loyalty to a brand

Figure 7.2 Brand Equity Pyramid

new customers. Organizations at the top, on the other hand, can count on brand loyalty for at least a portion of their customer base. Their marketing efforts will usually focus on reinforcing this loyalty and the brand's messages. These organizations must, of course, continue to meet the needs of their customers if they are not to be overtaken by an aggressive competitor working its way up the pyramid.

The tools to build brand identity include the brand name, logo, symbols, slogan, color, and graphic presentation.

Brand Name

A new imaging facility or one that seeks to change its identity will need to devise a brand name. Traditionally, healthcare organizations selected relatively generic names, often based on the names of the providers (eg, Smith Radiology Center) or geographic location (Chicago Hospital). While not necessarily negative, from a branding perspective, such names contribute little to differentiate the provider from its competitors or to build positive associations in the mind of consumers.

Ideally, a brand name will accomplish some of the following:

- Suggest product/service attributes or benefits (eg, AccuImaging)
- Be easy to pronounce, recognize, and remember

- Be distinctive
- Possess positive connotations in meaning, pronunciation, and visualization among all key consumer groups (including those for whom English is a second language)
- Engender positive associations among consumers
- Suggest organizational values
- Bring to mind the kinds of people who would buy the service
- Offer potential for growth (eg, satellite offices, new products)
- Be legally acceptable and available to be trademarked for protection

Given the substantial investment and long-term commitment to a brand name, choosing one should not be done in haste or without considerable thought and research. A substantial list of alternatives, based on the above attributes, should be collected and considered, then narrowed down to five to ten finalists. These should be researched for trademark status (by consulting an intellectual property attorney or the US Patent and Trademark Office). The finalists should be tested with focus groups or consumer surveys to ensure that only intended associations are generated. From a practical standpoint, the name should lend itself to creative representation and, if necessary, work with existing signage.

Logo and Symbols

The way in which the name is represented (in color and typeface) can be sufficiently distinctive as to negate the need for an accompanying logo or symbol. However, adding a logo or symbol can further build brand awareness, elicit positive associations, and differentiate the organization from its competitors.

Whereas logos are generally abstract designs, symbols can range from human spokespeople to representations of objects. A pediatric imaging facility might, for example, use a teddy bear as its symbol.

An effective logo or symbol will stand out from the competitors', contribute to the positive brand image, make the brand memorable, and appeal visually to not only those in the organization but also key target audiences. It will reproduce well in both large formats (eg, signage) and small (eg, business cards) and in both black and white and color. It will need to have visual impact when reproduced in newspapers and on the organization's Web site.

Slogan

Of all the branding tools, a slogan is probably the least essential. Nevertheless, "The effect of using the same slogan over and over again is almost hypnotic and subliminal in the brand image it creates."[3] As with a logo, a slogan becomes part of the graphic identity of the brand and appears whenever and wherever the brand name does.

A slogan may be as concise as a two word phrase or a slightly longer six word sentence. It should be memorable, meaningful to the target audiences, and associated with one or more positive attributes of the brand. If an agency is hired to create the organization's logo, it may also offer assistance in creating a slogan. Alternatively, involving staff in a brainstorming session would serve to stimulate interest in and support for the branding project. As with the brand name, once a list of potential slogans is generated, it should be culled to fewer than five. These should be verified that they are not already trademarked and tested with consumer focus groups or surveys before a finalist is selected. This process should be carried out in conjunction with the brand name and logo development whenever possible because the three elements will need to be incorporated into a single brand identity and design and the overall cost should be lower.

Unlike the brand name and logo, a slogan is subject to more frequent replacement either because it fails to add to brand identity or has become dated. On the other hand, slogans that become etched in consumers' minds can endure for many years.

Graphic Representation and Colors

With brand name, logo, and slogan determined, the final tool will provide the "glue" that will hold them together. Probably the single most important step an organization can take to build brand identity is the choice of specific colors in the graphic representation, crucial to presenting the brand consistently.[4] Color and graphics contribute to the brand's appeal, make it memorable, and help it stand out from the competition.

The selection of one or more colors for branding representation goes far beyond someone's favorite color. Anyone responsible for creating and maintaining a brand needs to keep color-related issues such as these in mind:

- Flexibility of use: Print and Internet reproduction will range from black-and-white newspaper advertisements to full color Web site postings. Generally, the selection of at least one color that is black or another very dark color provides the greatest readability when the brand must appear small and the greatest flexibility for subsequent design uses.
- Reproduction considerations: If forms or other items are regularly photocopied, a colored version of the brand should be tested for reproducibility before a final selection. If the facility prints its forms one at a time from the computer, printing the brand in the "official" colors will require a color printer. The more colors used, the more ink cartridges used (and the greater the cost). The use of color

affects costs for professional printing as well. Colors other than black cost more to print and the more colors used, the greater the cost.

- Psychological impact: Colors have different meanings in different cultures. Facilities that serve ethnic populations should carry out focus groups or other research to ensure the colors selected will not have unintended messages.

Graphic representation refers to the typeface, the fonts, and placement of the various branding elements. As with color, typefaces have personalities and engender associations that must be considered. Typefaces and fonts also have varying levels of readability. In most cases, the typeface selected for branding will also be used for other text on a document, so selecting a typeface that is widely available and highly readable in various sizes is essential. Web sites and other online media put special demands on the readability of a typeface, so it is wise to test the brand in these media.

The logo designer will make recommendations for color, type, and element placement, incorporating various options into a number of designs from which to select. Once a final design is chosen, the designer should prepare a master style sheet, or graphics standards, that will guide all future uses of the brand. It should specify the colors, typefaces, and fonts that can be used and how the elements relate to each other including relative spacing and placement on a page. This document should be accessible to all staff responsible for preparing any documents related to the brand, and its use should be reinforced with an in-service session on branding. No exceptions to the graphics standards should be allowed, in order to build brand awareness and equity.

Develop Communication Objectives

A key element of a marketing program is a marketing plan that outlines the overall goal(s) and objectives. What links the marketing objectives to the actual tactics used are the communication objectives. Generally, these spell out how marketing communications will influence the purchasing behavior of one or more target audiences. The following is a purchasing decision model with six stages, any one of which can be the focus of a communication objective[1]:

1. **Awareness:** Before consumers decide to make a purchase from a specific provider, they must be aware of both the provider and the desired behavior (eg, if a physician, refer patients). If the majority of the target audience has little or no awareness of an imaging facility, its services, or the behavior sought, then the communication objectives must first aim to build awareness.
2. **Knowledge:** Consumers can be aware of a product and/or a provider without knowing much about it. An individual may have heard of MRI, but without any

knowledge about what it is or why it is useful, he or she will not know how it might meet specific needs, perhaps even after consultation with a referring physician. Communication objectives will seek to increase the target audience's knowledge by transmitting key information.

3. **Positive association:** Consumers must have a favorable view of the provider and/or its services before they will consider a purchase. If market research shows a target audience has negative feelings about using a particular imaging facility, the reasons must be identified; any inadequacies of the facility must be corrected before a communications program can begin. Then its goal is to inform the target audience about the improvements.
4. **Preference:** At this stage, consumers know about the facility, understand its services, recognize how the facility would meet their needs, and have a favorable opinion. Nevertheless, their preference is for another facility, service, or behavior to meet their need. Communication must increase preference by promoting the facility's quality, performance, convenience, and other attributes.
5. **Conviction:** Despite having a preference, consumers may lack conviction to make the decision to act. A woman may have a positive opinion of a particular facility, may understand that mammography is safe and can be useful to detect breast cancer, but may lack conviction that she can benefit. The communication objectives would aim to build conviction about the value of mammography to her.
6. **Action:** Having worked through the five preceding steps, some consumers will still fail to act. Continuing the status quo is often perceived as easier than making a change; the consumer may plan to take action at a later date; or circumstances may interrupt the purchase decision process. Communication will generally concentrate on providing some incentive to act such as urging consumers to have an examination performed before the end-of-year expiration of medical benefits.

Because of the complexity of the healthcare purchasing decision-making process, the ability of marketing communications to directly influence the various target audiences can be difficult to identify and track. Usually, marketing communications focus on moving the target audience one stage at a time, rather than from stage 1 to stage 6. In healthcare, circumstances may intervene to preempt the process (eg, a man at stage 2 may develop symptoms that move him to stage 6).

As with marketing and other objectives, communications objectives should be clear, concise statements of what is to be accomplished and how; include a timeframe; be measurable; be ethical and legal; and be appropriate for the target audience. A single marketing objective may have several communication objectives. As an example, a facility is adding endovenous laser therapy for varicose veins to its interventional radiology services. One of its marketing objectives is to build awareness among the

35 referring physician practices with a goal of six referrals within the first 6 months. Among its communications objectives to achieve this are:

- Build awareness and knowledge among at least 30% of referring physicians by having a radiologist present a case review at the local hospital within 60 days of implementation, and by developing a short PowerPoint presentation that is used during brief individual meetings with representatives of at least 50% of practices within 30 days.
- Educate patients and physicians by developing custom pages linked to the facility's Web site, to be live from the first day the service is available.
- Drive traffic to the Web site and participation in the other activities by sending a brief e-mail message to all 35 practices on the first day the new procedure is available.

Identify Resources

Despite well crafted goals and objectives, the best plan will fail if adequate and appropriate resources are unavailable. These resources include more than money, although it is unlikely a marketing effort can be carried out without at least some financial investment. Before a marketing program can be implemented, a full assessment of available resources should be conducted, starting with an audit of existing marketing communications materials.

Audit Existing Marketing Materials and Activities

Nearly all healthcare organizations have at least some existing marketing communications materials and conduct some marketing activities, among them:

- Web site and other online marketing (eg, e-mail newsletters)
- Patient brochures and direct mail items (eg, newsletter)
- Patient amenities (eg, gowns)
- Signage, posters
- Stationery, business cards, forms
- Advertising
- Public relations
- Special events, including physician education seminars, health fairs, and community presentations

It may be tempting to continue to use existing items because doing so would save money and be easier, but this temptation should be resisted. Even existing materials and activities have a cost, such as staff time to make community presentations, which may take limited resources away from new elements that may accomplish objectives more effectively. All existing materials and activities should be carefully evaluated in relation to the marketing plan by asking whether they:

1. Present a message consistent with that of the plan
2. Address the target audience(s) sought
3. Have a history of effectiveness
4. Present the brand consistent with that of the plan
5. Achieve one or more of the communications objectives

Create a spreadsheet summarizing the existing items that will contribute to the new program to ensure that as the plan is implemented, these items will be effectively incorporated and no duplication will occur. The summary should include the type of item, quantity or frequency, resources needed to continue, target audience, key message(s), and objective met.

Identify Staffing Resources

For many healthcare organizations, locating the "who" will be harder than working out the "what" when it comes to implementing a marketing program. A hospital-based imaging department or an imaging center that is part of a large healthcare system may have access to a professional marketing staff. However, the imaging service may be just one of several vying for marketing assistance from these professionals, so there is the challenge of justifying priority status.

Marketing staff aside, few healthcare organizations have employees with unfilled work hours in which to carry out many of the activities incorporated in a marketing program. Therefore, before plans are finalized, explore all available avenues for staffing resources to implement the marketing plan. For example, it may be relevant to consider utilizing volunteers. Nonprofit healthcare organizations have long acknowledged the benefits of using volunteers to augment staff. Even a for-profit facility may be able to leverage the marketing talents of volunteers by establishing a Marketing Advisory Board or adding one or members with marketing expertise to its Board of Directors.

Hire Expertise

Even when a facility has success in acquiring donated services or finding volunteers or staff members to implement components of a marketing program, it may make sense to hire professionals as well. Among those who can contribute valuable expertise to a marketing program are:

Full-service marketing agencies: These companies provide all the services needed to carry out a marketing campaign, from research to creation to evaluation. These services may be provided by subcontractors, with the agency serving as "general contractor." The cost for this "one-stop shopping" can be substantial, as fees cover the agency's considerable overhead, mark-ups on subcontractor fees and material costs, and profit.

Specialized agencies: Many firms offer one or more marketing services, including advertising or public relations agencies, market research companies, Web site designers, and telemarketers. A specialist may be used for the most critical part of the program or to fill gaps in staff or volunteer expertise. While overall program costs will probably be lower than with a full-service agency, a substantial amount of time will be spent coordinating the various providers.

Individual consultants: Copy writers, designers, event planners, public relations professionals, photographers, media buyers (advertising), and focus group facilitators are just a few of the entrepreneurs who can be called on to carry out a specific task. The best among them will bring specialized training, experience from working for larger firms, flexibility, customer responsiveness, and a relatively low fee structure.

For tips on choosing and working with marketing agencies and consultants, see Box 7.1.

Identify Financial Resources

The budget prepared as part of the marketing plan provides the basis for the level of financial resources that will be needed. Ideally, the organization's revenues will be sufficient to cover the projected marketing expenses, especially if the marketing program is expected to generate additional revenues in the immediate term. Most programs will be implemented over a period of time, so at least some expenses can be budgeted into the future. A careful review of the organization's overall operating budget may reveal surpluses or costs that could be reduced or delayed to free up funds for the marketing program. If not, other financial resources, such as loans or fundraising, should be evaluated.

In 2008 an estimated $21.6 billion was given to healthcare organizations.[5] Four primary donor groups account for most of these funds: individuals, foundations, corporations, and government.

- **Individual Giving:** Individual giving is consistently the largest component of charitable contributions (comprised 75% of total giving in 2008[5]). Appeals are more effective when they ask for support of promising programs, rather than simply because an organization is needy or worthwhile. If wealthy individuals are approached one on one, the organization's representative should have a

Box 7.1 Choosing and Working with a Marketing Consultant

Using an advertising or public relations consultant (or agency) can be a cost-effective way to achieve marketing communications goals. An experienced consultant brings knowledge and skills based on working with similar clients, best practices that an administrator is unlikely to be familiar with, an outside perspective, and credibility in the eyes of senior management. The consultant will have access to multiple vendors, such as designers and writers, and may be better able to judge their suitability for a particular project. Here are some suggestions for selecting and working with communication consultants:

1. Know what is needed. Have goals and objectives in place, or at least define the problem or issue that the consultant will address.
2. Match the consultant to the task. Senior consultants may have experience in both advertising and public relations, but their fees will be commensurate with that experience.
3. Become familiar with the types of clients the prospective consultant has worked with. The more healthcare experience the consultant has, the easier it will be to bring the consultant up to speed on the facility.
4. Check references, review portfolios, and understand the types of services available.
5. Once a consultant has been selected, create a contract that clearly outlines responsibilities, time lines, finances, and expectations.
6. Educate the consultant. No matter how experienced the consultant is, he or she cannot know too much about the imaging facility. Provide copies of annual reports, current facility literature, organizational charts, and other basic documents to aid in planning and analysis. Put the consultant on the facility's distribution list for key documents.
7. Communicate with the consultant. Make sure objectives and expectations are clearly stated. Ask questions. Express concerns.
8. Be clear about who the contact person is, who will make the final decisions on all work produced by the consultant, and who must be included in all reviews.
9. Be responsive. Return calls, review submitted materials by the date agreed on (or negotiate a new date), and provide requested information in a timely fashion.
10. Respect the consultant and avoid second-guessing the advice. This relationship works most effectively when both parties recognize their individual strengths and weaknesses.

Source: Marquez LO. Marketing communications. In: Kroken P, Richardson E, Stockburger W, eds. *Communication & Information Management in Radiology*. Sudbury, MA: AHRA; 2007.

proposal prepared that follows the guidelines described above for soliciting services from businesses.

- **Foundations:** In 2008 more than 71,000 U.S. grant-making foundations gave away an estimated $41.2 billion, or 13% of total giving.[5] These organizations are comprised of (1) family foundations, established by wealthy individuals to support a limited number of activities; (2) general foundations, run by professionals and making grants for a wide range of activities globally; (3) corporate foundations, set up by large corporations to direct monetary gift giving without involving company officers; and (4) community foundations, entities that pool the funds of many smaller foundations and other private sources to lower administrative costs and increase the impact of grantmaking.[1] See Box 7.2.

Box 7.2 Grant-Making Resources

One of the best resources for locating appropriate foundations is the nonprofit Foundation Center, founded in 1956 to provide research and information on grant-making organizations and to connect nonprofits with grant opportunities. It regularly publishes various directories and a bibliography of state foundation directories is also available on its Web site.

The US Department of Health and Human Services has set up a Web-based portal that makes accessing the wide variety of granting agencies simple. It provides links to all U.S. government grant programs. Federal small business financing is the focus of Business.Gov, which provides links to state program information as well. Other resources may include state or local offices of economic development and the local chambers of commerce.

- **Corporations:** Businesses, with and without foundations, may also make donations of cash or in-kind goods and services. About 5% ($14.5 billion) of total giving in 2008 came from corporations, not including in-kind donations.[5] A request for donations from a corporation has the greatest likelihood of success when the prospects are local to the donor, and have related activities, expressed interests, personal relationships, and specific capabilities.[1]
- **Government:** Government agencies at local, state, and national levels can be a fruitful source of grant funding. It is possible to receive more than one grant from more than one agency simultaneously. As with foundations, research to identify agencies with a match to the imaging facility's interests and project is an important first step. Given that many government grants come with substantial requirements, these expectations should be reviewed and carefully evaluated for potential impact on the facility before an application is made. See Box 7.2.

Evaluate Promotional Options

This could be considered a golden time for marketers, as never before have there been so many ways to reach out to consumers, often in very targeted ways. However, at a time when virtually everyone is subject to "overcommunication" via Internet advertising, handheld computing, e-mail, and traditional media, it has become more difficult to determine the best combination and intensity of media to stimulate the desired results.

Selection Variables

Each marketing tactic has advantages and disadvantages (as shown in Table 7.1) as well as specific criteria by which to choose from among the alternatives.

Table 7.1 Comparison of Media for Healthcare Marketing

Media Option	*Strengths*	*Weaknesses*	*Considerations*
Newspaper	Can present detailed information Reaches older audience Short lead time High reach potential Immediate impact	Poor reach to younger audience Cluttered environment Very short lifespan Poor production values Few readers per copy	Production quality constrains design options
Magazine	Can present detailed information Pass-along readership expands reach High production values Upscale markets Association with editorial content provides credibility Long shelf life	Long lead time Relatively costly Less immediate impact on objective Lower reach	Requires longer term approach to campaign planning
Radio	Low cost per contact Segmentation of audience Short lead time Variable scheduling Local personalities available	High total cost for good reach Cluttered environment Audio impact only One exposure/expenditure Declining listenership, especially with younger audiences	Difficult to write memorable copy
Television	Audio and video presentation of message Immediate impact Schedule when needed Segmentation of audience possible	Costly to produce quality spot Message limited by commercial length Simple message Cluttered environment One exposure/expenditure Reach far beyond market in many areas	Production values must reflect quality
Outdoor advertising	Large reach Geographic concentration Low cost per exposure locally Flexible scheduling	Severely restricted message length No demographic selectivity Minimum purchase	Design is critical, especially visual impact
Direct mail/ brochures	Can present detailed information Demographic selectivity Relatively low cost in quantity Easy to track response Timing flexibility Can be personalized	Must have distribution plan Easy for target to discard/ ignore Visual impact only	Educational opportunity Cost per piece decreases with quantity ordered May be kept or passed along, expanding reach

Web-based media	Detailed content in some forms Near total control over content High audience involvement	Clear navigation, visual impact essential Cluttered environment User control over access Frequent content updates	User must be computer savvy Technological changes rapidly occur Must evaluate options for faddishness
Specialty items	Name and brand visibility Popular with most recipients	Severely restricted message length Cluttered environment Hard to measure impact Must have distribution plan	Functional items are kept, passed along Quality must reflect facility

This section focuses on selection variables that apply to all tactical options, including:

- Target audience reach
- Appropriateness for audience and message
- Suitability for the product or service
- Market environment
- Cost

Traditional Promotional Options

Despite the prevalence of high-technology options, most healthcare marketing programs utilize the traditional promotional tactics of advertising, public relations, and educational marketing and community outreach. Among the reasons these remain popular are: (1) they each have strengths that meet specific needs and achieve specific objectives; (2) they are flexible in application; (3) they can be implemented successfully by nonspecialists; and (4) they are compatible with healthcare culture.

Advertising

As healthcare facilities have recognized the potential for direct-to-consumer promotion, advertising has become the basis for many of their marketing programs. It comprises a wide range of media and formats including:

- **Newspapers:** The strength of newspaper advertising is its flexibility to display a relatively complex message, including details of location and operating hours. The greatest challenge lies in creating a design that can be easily seen and will capture the attention of the target market.
- **Magazines:** Because of their long lead times for advertising placement and production, messages may become quickly outdated. On the other hand, magazines tend to remain available to readers for a much longer time than many other media, increasing the reach.

- **Radio:** The cost per spot will be higher at radio's prime times, but listenership is also highest, so costs on a per-impression basis could actually be lower than at less expensive time periods. People are relatively habitual in their radio listening habits, increasing the likelihood that the same listeners will hear a message multiple times during a campaign.
- **Television:** Television advertising can be affordable locally on a per-impression basis. Spots can be purchased from local stations or on a localized basis from a cable company.
- **Direct mail:** Sending unsolicited material can be an effective tool for building and keeping brand awareness, collecting names for the facility's marketing database, and generating business. The right mailing list is one of the crucial elements in achieving this; the closer the match to the target audience, the greater the response rate. Direct mail allows a longer message than some other media, but the presentation must be compellingly written, well designed, and eye catching.
- **Outdoor advertising:** In nearly all cases, outdoor advertising (eg, billboards, signs, and bus/taxi cards) must be read within a few seconds, often from a distance. These media are suitable for very simple messages and because most signs will be seen repeatedly by thousands, outdoor advertising can be useful to build brand and image awareness.
- **Premiums:** Also known as specialty items or incentives, premiums comprise a wide range of imprintable, tangible items (eg, mugs, note pads, pens and pencils, T-shirts, tote bags, bumper stickers). These items can be used to attract attention to an accompanying offer or activity, build brand awareness and goodwill, and provide an incentive to action.
- **Web-based:** These programs will be discussed later in this chapter.

While a few media allow for relatively long messages, advertising tends to work best when messages are short. Most formats need photographs or other elements of visual interest and creativity to take those messages beyond the clutter of competing advertisements (Sidebar 7.1). Unless a response mechanism (eg, a coupon) is built into the advertising, however, a marketer may find evaluating effectiveness difficult, at least in the short term.

One key to an effective advertising campaign is repetition. Greater frequency is required when (1) the product is new, (2) the message is complex, (3) competitors advertise heavily, (4) the goal is to attract new consumers, (5) the marketing campaign is new, or (6) a special event is being promoted.[2] A multimedia campaign allows for repetition of a message in various media, each of which should reinforce the others. The successful media plan utilizes the strengths of different media options, referred to as the media mix, to present repetition of a consistent message in different ways to the broadest audience.

SIDEBAR 7.1: Components of a Great Printed Advertisement

Headline: Large-print words, usually at the top of the page, to attract the eye
Subhead: Slightly smaller print addition to headline that provides details (optional)
Body copy: Main text, set in readable size and typeface, written clearly and concisely
Visual: Photograph or illustration for visual impact (optional, but preferable)
Caption: Brief text to explain visual (optional)
Logo and signature: Trademarked version of the business name, incorporating the specific typeface, color(s), and graphics that identify the brand
Slogan: Brief phrase representative of the brand identity (optional)
White space: Blank space in and around advertisement's copy, which draws the reader's attention and is vastly underrated by non-designers

Source: Hiam A. *Marketing for Dummies*. 3rd ed. Hoboken, NJ: Wiley Publishing; 2009:116–117.

Public Relations

Public relations seeks to positively affect attitudes toward and build awareness of a product or organization among not only consumers, but also regulators, legislators, funders, business leaders, managed care administrators, and employees. It can be useful to build brand awareness, influence decision makers, introduce a new service, and inform the public about health issues. Its primary tactic is publicity, which seeks to generate unpaid media coverage via tools such as:

- News releases
- Feature stories
- Editorials, opinion pieces, and letters to the editor
- Public service announcements on television and radio
- Talk show appearances
- Public event appearances
- Online forums and blogs

The stories generated by publicity efforts tend to be viewed by the public at large in a more positive light and as more objective than paid advertising. However, coverage is largely in the control of the media, with no guarantees that a marketer's efforts will result in actual stories. Furthermore, although the coverage is unpaid, conducting a public relations campaign still has costs in terms of staff time and often consultant fees. Before marketers decide to include publicity in a marketing plan, they should ask the following questions[2]:

1. Do the objectives, marketing strategies, and issue lend themselves well to publicity?

2. Does the organization need and want the added dimension of legitimacy that public relations brings to the overall communications effort?
3. Does the organization need the additional media impact (without media spending), knowing coverage is uncertain?
4. Is the organization willing to make the investment to attempt to generate publicity? How likely is it that the investment will be worth it?

News releases are probably the single most important component of a publicity campaign, as they may not only be printed as is by a newspaper, but also generate feature stories and editorials written by journalists and requests to appear on talk shows or at special events. Releases can also be repurposed for different audiences (eg, posted on the organization's Web site or abridged and published in its newsletter).

"Consistent, high-quality news release content brands a company or nonprofit as a busy market player, an active expert in the industry, and a trusted resource to turn to."[6] Producing releases with high-quality content that meets journalists' needs and distributing the documents appropriately substantially increase the likelihood of coverage. In general, an effective release is timely; is written accurately, clearly, and concisely, without jargon; and has a degree of novelty. The release should lead with the basics—the "who, what, where, when, and why"— in a format that objectively presents information and is not self-congratulatory or editorializing. The final paragraph will usually be similar for all releases and include generic information about the organization, its services, and how readers can contact it. The overall length should be kept to two pages or less; optional addenda include a high-quality photograph with caption, a one page background sheet, or a one page fact sheet with key message points.

Many organizations tend to underestimate their newsworthiness, especially to local media. They wait for the "big story," focus on hard-to-reach regional and national media, and miss numerous opportunities to use their expertise to inform the public and build awareness (Box 7.3). Compile a list of editors and/or reporters who cover business, healthcare, and special events within their service area. Releases should be sent via e-mail to appropriate media outlets and only rarely to the entire list. Online services are also available to distribute releases on a regional basis for a fee.

For more about writing and distributing public relations materials, see AHRA's book *Communication & Information Management in Radiology*.

Educational Marketing and Community Outreach

Educational marketing and community outreach activities have a long and successful history in healthcare. The strategies are applicable to various target audiences

Box 7.3 Making News

While not everything happening at an imaging facility is worthy of a press release, many fail to fully appreciate and take advantage of the range of possible news items. Here is just a sampling suitable for local media coverage:

- **Staff related**: Promotions, additions, election to professional association posts, honors and awards, papers published, conference presentations, completion of specialized training
- **Service related**: Changes in hours, new locations, programs or services added, new technology additions, reopening after renovations
- **Activities**: Open house, participation in health fair, special screening programs, public seminars or physician presentations, public events for special months (eg, Breast Cancer Awareness Month), charitable donations or volunteer projects in the community
- **Business accomplishments**: Certifications, significant business goals achieved, special recognition, acquisition of another practice

and are a natural fit with the healthcare culture. Both the sponsor and the participants perceive value on several levels:

1. Educational literature and activities give the organization's marketing representatives reasons to call on referring physicians, their staffs, other business executives, or health plan administrators.
2. The activities help the organization establish itself as a trusted "expert" in the community.
3. Participants are better informed, often at little or no cost to themselves.
4. The organization gains visibility and awareness via a strategy that is usually perceived by recipients as less commercial and more objective than advertising.
5. Education topics lend themselves to the development of programs and materials that can be used in multiple tactics (eg, a live presentation videotaped and uploaded to the organization's Web site).

The opportunities to present educational messages are substantial, limited primarily by budget and staff to implement them. For referring physician groups, for example, topics could include new technologies and procedures available, getting the most from PACS, how they can best prepare their patients for a procedure, and case reports reflecting medical necessity issues. The tools to provide the educational message might include an open house for physicians and their staff, a Grand Rounds presentation, a physicians' newsletter or special section on the facility's Web site, a blog, or "lunch and learn" seminars. For patients, educational topics might include what to expect from a procedure, how the latest imaging technology is affecting diagnosis and treatment, how to prepare for a visit, and how the various subspecialties differ. Possible tools include a patient page with frequently asked questions on the facility's Web site, brochures available at referring physicians' offices, or a newsletter.

Community outreach takes an educational message to a broader audience. Hospital-based imaging departments and freestanding centers, for example, have long been involved in breast cancer awareness programs and events. Other possible activities include participating in a panel discussing current treatment options for varicose veins or appropriate use of ultrasound in prenatal care; conducting an open house to introduce new technology; distributing a health and wellness newsletter to the community at large; or offering tours for school groups.

Events may be conducted by the imaging facility itself; the organization may sponsor activities of other groups; or it may be a participant in another group's event. In assessing the suitability of an educational or community outreach event for the marketing program, it should be established that:

1. The connection between the event and the organization is clear and meaningful.
2. The facility's identity will be communicated clearly.
3. The event has a compelling appeal to the target audience.
4. The event lends itself to using existing communications materials or applying newly created items to achieve other marketing objectives.
5. At least one key goal can be established and the results measured.
6. Resources are available to carry out or participate in the event.
7. The event has at least local news value.

For more about conducting seminars and community events, see AHRA's book *Communication & Information Management in Radiology*.

Emerging Promotional Options

The traditional tools and strategies remain the basis of an effective marketing program for most imaging organizations. However, given the budget constraints and competitive challenges faced by healthcare marketers, less traditional options are being adopted when they meet specific marketing needs. Among these newer options are Web-based marketing, service line marketing, and social marketing.

Web-Based Marketing

The Internet is transforming marketing tactics, even for businesses that do not want to potentially reach millions of people. In fact, despite the massive numbers of participants overall, online media offer ideal venues for niche marketers who can appeal to only those who are searching for related content at any given moment.

Although newspapers and other traditional media have significant generational usage patterns, the Internet can potentially reach a wide range of audiences, including many of the most desirable patients. An estimated 52% of Americans aged 62 to 71, for example, are online with 38% of them searching for health-related information. They are twice as likely to be employed, have twice the annual income, and are more than one and a half times as likely to have attended college as those who do not use the Internet.[7]

At present, an imaging facility can use online media to carry out research; provide information in print, audio, and video formats; conduct discussion forums; and provide interactive training. From a marketing perspective, online media can build awareness, establish credibility and thought leadership, and promote services. Unlike retail and many other businesses, however, an imaging facility should plan to spend only a very small portion of its marketing budget on online tactics; some experts suggest no more than 1% to 2% of revenues.[4] As with traditional media, the marketer must choose from among the online media options based on the organization's marketing strategy and resources. The options include the organization's Web site; Web advertising; blogs; and social networking or social media (not to be confused with social marketing).

Web sites: An organization's Web site is the hub for all its online marketing. Marketers need to remember that great content is the most important aspect of any Web site. It will encourage visitors to stay on the site longer, return more often, forward useful content to others, and generally increase traffic to the site (see Box 7.4).

Two types of content are generally used: Durable content remains relevant for long periods and requires updating only about once a year; ephemeral content is time sensitive and may be useful for as little as a few days. In addition to basic information (eg, directions, contact information), other categories should be considered:

- Frequently asked questions (patient version and physician version)
- Descriptions of tests and treatments (patient version and physician version)
- Glossary of terms for lay readers
- Instructional videos for patients (eg, how to prepare for test) and scheduling staff
- Referring physician newsletter or blog on trends in radiology
- Patient newsletter or blog on health and wellness topics
- Careers page for prospective employees
- List of suggested reading; links to high-quality health Web sites
- Calendar and highlights of community outreach activities

Box 7.4 Search Engine Optimization Helps Searchers Find a Web Site

A simple online search can result in thousands of responses. The practice of making a Web site as visible as possible to Internet search engines is known as search engine optimization (SEO). Some techniques are used by the Web site designer, others by those who develop content, and still others by consultants specializing in SEO. Here are a few suggestions to boost the facility's site visibility:

1. The site designer should be sure to include a header block with a title element, not viewable on the page. The title should be specific about and unique to the page's content and have an H1 tag before and after it (a signal to the search engines).
2. The site designer should include META tags, which are lines of HTML code that identify the document properties and use keywords searchers are likely to use.
3. The site should have a well-designed site map, either as a descriptive navigation bar (for simple sites) or as a separate page. It should list all pages by title or topic and provide a direct link to each one.
4. Every Web presence for the facility (eg, Web site, blog, social media pages) should have consistent branding and strong usernames.
5. Efforts should be made to build traffic with current customers. The more traffic a site has, the higher the ranking on a search engine. The facility's Web site should be listed on all communications; content should be useful and encourage customers to return often.
6. The facility's Web site should include links to other professional and health information sites, especially those that are highly ranked on search engines. The higher ranked sites tend to bring up the ranking of sites linked to it.

Source: Hiam A. *Marketing for Dummies*. 3rd ed. Hoboken, NJ: Wiley Publishing; 2009.

- Media room, including archives of news releases, background information, annual report, photographs or video of key staff and facility, that may be useful to journalists and others
- Video or audio of staff presentations at professional meetings and community events

Beyond content, the core elements of a successful Web site include: (1) clear, simple navigation; (2) non-text content such as video clips and photographs; (3) feedback mechanisms (eg, easy-to-find and use "Contact us" information); and (4) a professional, consistent site personality that fits with the organization's brand.

Web advertising: As with other forms of Internet-based marketing, the options for advertising on the Web continue to expand. A marketer can choose to use pay-per-click advertisements on search engines, banner advertisements on Web sites, or variations of these in the form of buttons, half-banners, and "skyscrapers" (vertical banner ads). By carefully selecting the Web sites on which to advertise, it is possible to more closely match viewers with the target audience. Sites selected should be a good fit for the facility and its services (eg, a local women's spa). Some social media sites, for example, allow advertisers to target specific profiles according to age, gender, location, and other variables which will then receive a banner advertisement.

Pay-per-click advertising is offered by all Internet search engines. The advertiser creates a one-sentence description, links it to key terms the target audience would search for, and bids for the per-click price (which may be as low as 50 cents). The higher the bid, the closer to the top of the search page the advertisement appears. Each time a user clicks on the description, the advertiser owes the search engine company.

Deciding where to advertise is just the first step in the process of attracting customers via the Internet. The advertiser must also carefully plan where to send someone who clicks on a search engine listing or banner ad. Generally, a dedicated landing page (with a unique URL) is preferable to the facility's home page. A landing page can directly tie into the ad content and include some form of response mechanism (eg, call to action such as scheduling a mammography screening appointment or asking for additional information). All forms of Web advertising need to be kept extremely brief and eye-catching to increase effectiveness.

Blogs: Weblogs, known as blogs, are a special form of Web site, featuring an individual's opinions and comments on any topic. A marketing program can make use of blogs in several ways[6]:

1. To monitor what is being said about the organization, relevant markets, and the industry by reading key blogs regularly using specialized blog search engines
2. To participate in blog conversations by commenting on other people's blogs
3. To begin to affect content by submitting news releases to key bloggers and by creating and writing a blog

Reading other blogs can provide valuable market research and will help a potential blogger understand the unwritten rules and get a sense of what makes a blog work. Blog commentators and authors should be transparent (eg, use their own names); respect the privacy and confidentiality of the organization, its data, and its patients; disclose the business affiliation and any conflicts of interest; be truthful; and give credit when material from other sources is used.[6] If a marketer or other member of the facility's staff wants to start a blog, note the following[6]:

- The topic should be one the writer feels passionate about, will appeal to the target audience(s), and is relatively narrow.
- The tone should be authentic and appropriate to the audience.

- The look and feel should be in line with the facility's branding guidelines, but should be distinctive to signal "this is an independent voice."
- The name and tagline (slogan) will be indexed by search engines and will be very difficult to change later, so these items should be carefully planned.
- Blogging software makes the process of designing and creating blogs simple and relatively inexpensive. However, changing software is very difficult, so each software program should be carefully assessed before a final selection is made.
- Several options are available for the blog URL (Internet address). The blog can be mapped from the facility's domain name, it can have its own domain name, or it can have a URL through the blogging software.
- The blog should include a page of background—the writer's biography, credentials for writing the blog, and affiliations/conflicts of interest.

Social Networking: Given the meteoric rise in popularity of social networking Web sites, it is not surprising that marketers are looking for acceptable ways to reach the networked millions. These sites allow participants to create a profile and build virtual networks of individuals with similar interests, thereby presenting ready-made niches for marketers who can effectively tap into those interests. The sites appeal to different users, so a marketer should spend time on each site before posting any information.

Among the possible uses for social networks in a marketing program are to post the facility's blog with links to its Web site, thereby expanding its reach; post clips from community outreach activities (again with a link to the Web site) to build goodwill and awareness; and create a group with relevant professional interests, with whom to exchange market research, best practices, and resource referrals.

Service Line Marketing

Service line marketing is a natural complement to educational marketing, in that it tends to focus on educating consumers about the qualities that make a service line unique and special. The strategy is generally fact based and intellectual, especially in comparison to an organization's overall branding campaign, which may appeal more to consumers' emotions.

Physician expertise, technological developments, patient outcomes, and quality rankings are among the concepts around which service line marketing builds its messages, using the same tools as the overall marketing program. Many healthcare consumers are knowledgeable about health and wellness and are actively involved in the decisions surrounding their care. They expect providers to be open about their capabilities, the pros and cons of their services, and their qualifications to meet the consumers' specific needs. Service line marketing accommodates these intellectual expectations. On the other hand, marketers must be scrupulous in presenting accurate, verifiable information that does not mislead. The very qualities that make these consumers receptive to a service line message make them equally adept at accessing alternative information sources to verify claims.

Service line marketing can be a useful component of a marketing program, especially when a facility adds a service line, acquires technology or a radiologist that makes it a market leader in a given subspecialty, or decides to limit the practice to a narrow service line range. Although the messages will vary from those of a facility's overall program, a service line campaign must nevertheless clearly relate to it: use of logo, slogan, and other key design components should conform to the facility's branding standards. Consumers should never be confused about the fact that a given service line is a component of the imaging facility. In this way, the branding campaign benefits from the support of the service line campaign, which benefits from the credibility built by branding.

Social Marketing

Social marketing (not to be confused with social networking) differs from general marketing not in its tools, but in its objectives. Kotler and Andreasen, leaders in the field, have defined it as seeking "to influence *social behaviors* not to benefit the marketer but *to benefit the target audience and the general society*."[1] Thus, those involved in social marketing programs carry out planned efforts to influence a wide range of human behaviors for largely selfless reasons. For example, one or several imaging facilities might collaborate with the local chapter of the American Cancer Society to encourage women to undergo mammography with the goal of reducing morbidity and mortality from breast cancer within their community. While a facility may benefit if the women seek examinations, that is not the primary goal. In fact, the program might include an offer of free or reduced price examinations for qualified women in order to achieve the desired behavior.

Social marketing faces many challenges since behavior can be very difficult to change. Easiest to influence are one-time behaviors involving individuals such as convincing a pregnant woman to undergo ultrasound. Behaviors that are repetitive and call for a high degree of involvement (value-based) by groups are the toughest (eg, ending racial prejudice). Social marketers are also challenged by the fact that change may be hard to discern and long in coming, yet they must be able to demonstrate effectiveness. Other challenges include (1) the need to promote behaviors the target audience may not find agreeable, (2) excessive expectations, (3) issue sensitivity, (4) intangible consequences that are hard to describe, and (5) limited budgets.

SIDEBAR 7.2: Ten Tips for Successful Social Marketing

1. **Talk with and listen to customers.** The central focus of social marketing is meeting the needs and wants of customers.
2. **Segment the audience.** The more similar each group's members are, the more likely a message can be devised that will strike a cord with them.
3. **Position the product.** Positioning usually will be based either on the benefits or on the removal of barriers to making the change.
4. **Know the competition.** The marketing message must make the change being promoted more attractive than the alternatives.
5. **Go where the audience is.** Research must identify how the target audience gets its news and spends its free time.
6. **Use a variety of approaches.** Any of the many tools described in this chapter can be used; however, using an overarching look, logo, and slogan helps ensure campaign cohesion.
7. **Use models that work.** Look to behavioral sciences for basic models to guide strategies and audience segmentation.
8. **Test repeatedly.** To avoid wasting valuable resources, every component of a campaign should be tested with the target audience(s) to evaluate effectiveness.
9. **Build partnerships with key allies.** These partnerships can bring attention and credibility to the program, provide access to new audiences, and pool scarce resources.
10. **Evaluate the program and learn from mistakes.** Evaluation occurs throughout a program, guiding changes in strategy, tactics, or messages midstream if the desired action is not happening.

Source: Adapted from Weinreich NK. Building social marketing into your program. Available at: http://www.social-marketing.com/building.html. Accessed January 8, 2010.

Market research is essential at every phase of a social marketing campaign. These campaigns are customer driven, so it is important to understand just where the target audience stands on the issue before devising strategy. Interim research is necessary to test tactical alternatives, ensure messages are being perceived as intended, and evaluate progress. Social marketers recognize the need for flexibility and the need to change tactics, messages, or even the "product" in response to research (Sidebar 7.2).

Additional information on social marketing is available from the Social Marketing Institute in Washington, DC.

Conclusion

In the competitive healthcare industry, attracting and retaining customers can only be achieved through an effective marketing program. Implementing such a program is as important to organizational success as offering the latest technology and the best trained staff. Given the broad range of promotional options, focus is essential. By clearly defining the facility's position, brand, and the marketing communications goals, management is positioned to choose the best options within the available resources to achieve the desired goals, thus ensuring the viability of the organization.

References

1. Kotler P, Andreasen AR. *Strategic Marketing for Nonprofit Organizations.* Englewood Cliffs, NJ: Prentice Hall;1991.
2. Hiebing RG Jr, Cooper SW. *The One-Day Marketing Plan.* 2nd ed. Lincolnwood, IL: NTC Business Books; 1999.
3. Kotler P. *Kotler on Marketing: How to Create, Win, and Dominate Markets.* New York, NY: The Free Press;1999:63, 66.
4. Hiam A. *Marketing for Dummies.* 3rd ed. Hoboken, NJ: Wiley Publishing; 2009.
5. US charitable giving estimated to be $307.65 billion in 2008 [news release]. Glenview, IL: Giving USA Foundation; June 10, 2009. Available at: http://www.philanthropy.iupui.edu/News/2009/docs/GivingReaches300billion_06102009.pdf. Accessed January 19, 2010.
6. Scott DM. *The New Rules of Marketing and PR.* Hoboken, NJ: John Wiley & Sons; 2009:197–199.
7. We rule the net! *AARP The Magazine.* 2008; 51(5B):110.

Chapter 8

Evaluate the Marketing Program

J. Lynne Dodson and Luis O. Marquez

Implementing a marketing program without incorporating evaluation methodology means that invaluable data are lost to the organization—data that can be used to justify marketing expenses, plan future activities, correct operational deficiencies, and acknowledge employee contributions to the marketing effort. Marketers have a wide range of metrics from which to choose, based on the type of activities being carried out, the evaluation resources available, and how the results will be used. Evaluation tools range from spreadsheets to various types of financial analysis.

Evaluating a marketing program comprises monitoring the ongoing activities, evaluating their effectiveness and assessing their efficiency. As with other aspects of carrying out marketing within healthcare organizations, evaluation has its special challenges. One of the most significant is the impact of myriad factors on healthcare consumer behavior that are beyond the control of the organization. An imaging center may conduct an outstanding marketing campaign, but its effects are undermined if a major health plan changes its coverage or reimbursement rates fall.

Another challenge is the difficulty in defining success, and therefore measuring it, for some healthcare activities and their related marketing efforts. Many imaging facilities, especially those based in hospitals, must provide services that will never make a profit (eg, to uninsured or underinsured patients). As typical financial metrics are of little value in such instances, other measures must be used.

Measurement issues can also arise because healthcare services are often so interrelated that it is difficult to isolate the activities of one department and their effects. A mammography center that refers patients with positive test results to affiliated providers, for example, will probably want to find a way to measure this "extended impact" for its marketing campaign.

Reasons to Evaluate Marketing Activities

Despite the difficulties, no marketing initiative should be planned without incorporating evaluation activities throughout the process. Monitoring that deadlines and budgets are being met helps ensure that resources are used efficiently and that activities are carried out as planned. Setting and measuring interim outcome and impact goals allow the plan to be modified when necessary, enhancing the final results.

Evaluation provides valuable data for ongoing strategic planning as well. Organizations that are carrying out formal marketing activities for the first time gain baseline data against which to compare future actions. Experienced marketers get another set of data to track ongoing trends and/or changes within or beyond the organization.

Yet another reason to include evaluation in all marketing projects is the need to justify the expense both internally and externally. As reimbursement rates decline, the need increases to account for every dollar spent to senior management and, for nonprofit organizations, to foundations and other funding sources. As regulators and others seek to further reduce and control healthcare costs, every activity will be scrutinized; data will be needed that show increases in patients served, procedures carried out, awareness built, and other positive parameters that result from marketing efforts.

Finally, those who participate in marketing activities want and need to know that their efforts were worthwhile. Every employee will have a role in an imaging facility's marketing; some of them may have to learn new skills or carry out additional tasks; changes in patient load or characteristics may challenge workflow. Outcome and impact data reflect the contribution of the employees' efforts and offer information that can guide their future actions. Interim monitoring provides process data that give employees input on their current actions and help in prioritizing tasks.

Types of Evaluation

Healthcare marketing can be evaluated in at least three categories: process, outcome, and impact.[1] Process assessment evaluates the mechanics of the marketing campaign, especially tasks completed, deadlines met, roles performed, and content developed (ie, message consistency). For large scale projects in particular, process evaluation is essential for effective ongoing monitoring and to assess marketing efficiency.

In addition to the mechanics, process evaluation should attempt to assess issues such as:

- **Content:** Was the message conveyed clearly and consistently across the various activities (eg, the same key points emphasized in advertisements, at health fair displays, and by staff talking with patients)? Were readability and comprehension levels of communication materials appropriate for the target audience?
- **Components:** Were the various campaign activities effectively integrated, both in terms of how they were carried out and how they were perceived by the target audience? For example, if advertisements emphasized personal service, did staff meet patient expectations for service?
- **Reach:** To what extent was the target audience exposed to the campaign message? How well did the campaign reach the target audience without "scatter" to peripheral audiences?

The implementation plan serves as the basis for the process evaluation, as the plan sets out the timeline, tasks, distribution methods, and other process details. The metrics and tools used are described below.

Outcome evaluation assesses marketing effectiveness, that is, how well the activities changed behavior, attitudes, and preferences as specified in the goals and objectives. Many of the financial assessments (eg, changes in revenues, patient volume) are measures of outcome, but other issues serve to demonstrate effectiveness as well, such as:

- **Awareness:** How has awareness of the imaging facility and/or its services changed among members of the target audience? Have changes occurred relative to awareness of competitors?
- **Attitudes:** To what extent did levels of positive perception among the target audience change with regard to the organization as a whole or to specific services marketed during the campaign?
- **Knowledge:** How have depth and breadth of the target audience's knowledge changed with regard to the educational themes of the campaign (eg, diagnostic options for breast cancer)?

Impact evaluation, another means of assessing marketing effectiveness, seeks to determine whether the marketing campaign actually achieved the changes sought. This form of evaluation will generally be more relevant in social marketing campaigns that seek community-wide changes and is probably the most difficult to achieve accurately.[1] This is particularly true in healthcare, in which the impact may take many years to be revealed. A campaign that seeks to reduce deaths from breast cancer by encouraging mammograms, for example, can assess *outcome* by detecting changes in rates of mammograms performed. However, *impact* as measured by declining death rates is not likely to come from a single campaign nor will it occur within a short time after completion of the campaign. Some issues indicative of impact that may be relevant (and measurable) to campaigns conducted by imaging facilities include:

- **Lifestyle:** Have members of the target audience made relevant changes in their behavior and/or lifestyle?
- **Market share:** Has the facility's overall market share changed or its market position improved following the campaign?
- **Incidence:** Have relevant disease incidence rates changed within the target audience (especially in comparison to those of the community at large)?

Measurement Metrics and Tools

What tools and metrics do organizations use to determine whether marketing efforts have been successful? In some cases, results will be immediately evident in volume increases; in other instances, change will be more subtle or gradual. If marketing is carefully integrated with operations, measures of success will extend beyond a growth in the number of procedures performed. The bottom line, however, is that marketing efforts should produce measurable results.

While it is tempting to isolate various marketing or media tactics in order to evaluate their individual effectiveness, the strength of the marketing strategy is best measured cumulatively. Each element is important but each has strengths and weaknesses. Together, the various marketing options support each other, reinforce the message, and better facilitate action. Thus, to evaluate the success of most campaigns will require more than one tool and multiple metrics (Sidebar 8.1) with selection depending on the marketing goals and objectives, the tactics used, the budget, and available evaluation resources.

Measurement Tools

With increasing use of electronic medical records, the organization may already have systems in place to track the necessary data. With the project's goals and objectives as guides, a selection can be made from a variety of tools such as the following.

Pretests and posttests and surveys: Particularly useful in tracking changes in attitudes, behavior, and knowledge, tests and surveys can be administered to the entire target market or to a sample. These instruments should focus on the key parameters

SIDEBAR 8.1: Possible Evaluation Metrics

Financial Outcome Measures

- **Procedure volume:** Changes in total volume by: modality, referring physician or physicians group, payer; comparisons made short term or over multiple years
- **Revenue:** Changes in revenue for the entire system or by: department, procedure code, modality, referring physician or group, payer; comparisons made short term or over multiple years
- **Ratios:** Facility sales as a percentage of total sales in the target market (market share); actual cost versus budget (for individual components and for campaign as a whole); cost per sales call/cost per sale (for referring physicians); cost per response (or cost per new patient) for direct mail or sales promotion (eg, exhibits at health fairs); total marketing expense versus total sales

Customer Outcome Measures

- **Satisfaction:** Scheduling parameters (eg, rate of telephone response, appointment wait); registration parameters (eg, simplicity, speed); insurance plans offered; access to radiologist for consultation; report turnaround time; report accuracy; technology (eg, referring physician access to picture archiving and communication system)
- **Problem resolution:** Types of problems and their impact on facets of the operation (eg, work flow, compliance, customer service); time to resolution
- **Retention:** Numbers/percentages of repeat customers (referring physicians and patients) and new customers; rate of change over previous years
- **Attitudes and perceptions:** Expressed awareness and positive perception of facility's services, and preference for using them

Process Measures

- **Public relations:** Number of press releases distributed, press inquiries, and incidences and/or inches of media coverage
- **Advertising:** Number of placements and deadlines met; size of target audience reached; consumer recall; response to advertisement offer (eg, free breast self-exam guide)
- **Sales:** Numerical data reflecting responses by referring physicians and third party payers: office calls logged; visits made; contacts at exhibit (eg, local business or health expo); promotional literature pieces distributed; number and/or size of contracts finalized
- **Community relations:** Number of events and participants; level of awareness; participant recall of content
- **Direct marketing:** Amount of pieces distributed and deadlines met; number of responses; sum of patients generated

Impact Measures

- **Behavior:** Rate of change in behavior (focus of marketing) within target audience
- **Incidence/prevalence:** Change of disease (focus of marketing) rate within target audience compared to community at large
- **Market share:** Change in facility market share within target market

the project aims to change. Presumably, differences in results reflect the effect of marketing.

Interviews: Members of the target audience can be interviewed in person or by telephone to measure satisfaction and related marketing goals. Staff members can be interviewed with regard to their marketing roles and other process metrics.

Observation: Observation carried out by a trained evaluator can provide first-hand data, especially related to behavior, attitudes, and knowledge. For example, staff could be observed as they perform specified marketing tasks to assess factors related to efficiency and effectiveness, or patients could be observed to establish whether key learning objectives were achieved.

Media tracking: A spreadsheet can be used to track the number of press releases sent, level of coverage, and other marketing communications metrics within a specified time period. These data can be analyzed by comparing them with other periods and with project goals and objectives.

Sales trend analysis: By analyzing trends in key financial metrics (eg, revenues or the number of patients served), the effect of the marketing project can be evaluated on the facility's growth. One method calls for the calculation of metrics for different time frames: a given period before a test of the marketing activities (pretest), a comparable period as the test is being carried out (test), and a similar period following completion of the test during implementation of the full marketing project (posttest). Comparing pretest and test results demonstrates the likely impact of the project; comparing test and posttest results indicates any ongoing effect for the marketing activities; and comparing pretest and posttest results offers a longer term assessment of the marketing project's effectiveness.[2] Applying a growth rate improvement analysis such as the one shown in Table 8.1 provides additional insight into the long-term effects of the marketing activities.

As customer satisfaction encompasses a number of important metrics for many marketing activities, all of the tools discussed in Chapter 11 should be considered marketing tools as well.

Putting Evaluation Data to Work

Successful healthcare organizations recognize the wealth of operational information that can be mined from the results of marketing evaluation. Here are two examples of ways to evaluate marketing activities and put the resulting data to work to effectively meet customers' needs and wants.

Table 8.1 Example of Growth Rate Improvement Analysis

	No. procedures Previous year	*No. procedures Current year*	*% change*
Preperiod (4/6–5/2)			
Two test sites	2850	3125	10
System wide	6000	6475	8
Test period (5/4–6/1)			
Two test sites	2700	3070	14
System wide	5500	5800	5
Growth rate improvement (GRI)	*Preperiod % change*	*Test period % change*	*% point gain (loss)*
Two test sites	10	14	+4
System wide	8	5	−3
% point difference	2	9	+7[a]

[a] Incremental volume (GRI): 7% × 3070 test period volume = 215 net weekly gain

Source: Adapted from Hiebing RG Jr, Cooper SC. *The One-Day Marketing Plan*. 2nd ed. Lincolnwood, IL: NTC Business Books; 1999:307.

Case Study Example: New Computed Tomography Services

Quality Imaging decided to update its computed tomography (CT) scanner and focus on promoting those services to a target audience comprised of physician groups that had previously referred patients for CT examinations. The imaging facility's marketing representative visited each of the key practices, meeting with a physician and scheduling staff member. The messages conveyed by the marketing representative included highlights of the scanner's new applications particularly relevant to the practice—the device's improved capabilities that shortened examination times and added more scheduling slots each day. In terms of the "What's in it for me?" message, the representative emphasized the increased convenience for prompt scheduling and related report turnaround times, which would allow the referring physicians to expedite diagnosis and treatment of their patients' conditions, thereby increasing their patient satisfaction and comfort. During the first few weeks following installation, the scheduling staff called the target practices to inform them of the availability of short notice openings as a method to fill available capacity.

The new CT unit was put in place in May, and the facility tracked overall volume trends throughout the year. Their metrics shown in Figure 8.1 tracked a steady increase from June to August. In October, they began offering services on Saturday mornings, and it was evident volume again increased. As this example demonstrates, tracking by modality or in regard to overall volume is one of the options for measuring marketing efforts.

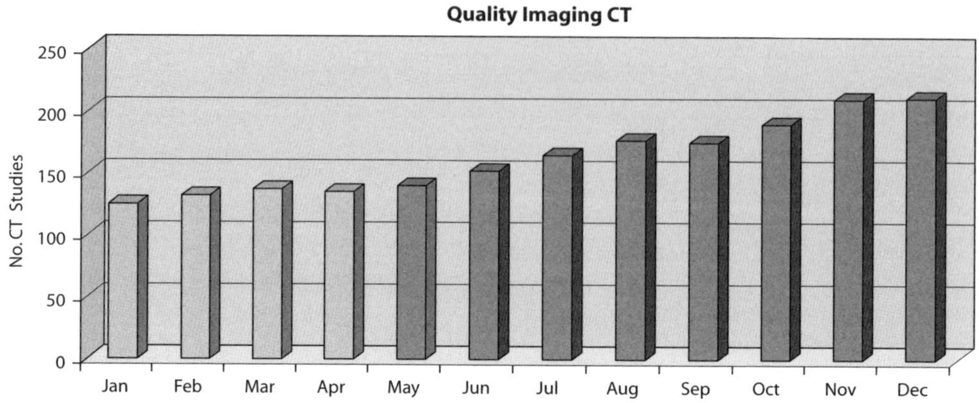

Figure 8.1 Quality Imaging CT Volume Trends

Case Study Example: Referring Physician Trends

Northside Hospital, including its imaging department, has an active marketing program, with a focus on physician education and problem resolution. Referrals by key practices are closely monitored on a monthly basis, including referrals both by the overall group and by its individual physicians. Marketing representatives quickly respond to declines in volume and revenue. In some cases, they discover a referring physician was on vacation during the month, explaining the decline in the rate of procedure requests. In other instances, a service problem had occurred, in which case a marketing staff member follows up with the referring physician to ensure the problem has been resolved to the physician's satisfaction. If necessary, marketing staff meet with the imaging administrator to plan staff education and/or institute process changes to ensure the problem does not recur.

Table 8.2 presents data on the referrals by individual physicians of the Northeast Multispecialty Group and details the action steps taken as information was tracked and analyzed.

Northside Hospital's imaging department also tracks referral totals for key groups (Figure 8.2); results are reviewed monthly. Changes in overall referral patterns are used to evaluate service/operational issues, determine the potential demand for new procedures, and evaluate the need for additional marketing activities.

Conclusion

A well-designed strategic marketing program should produce measurable results, which will be invaluable in assessing the effectiveness and efficiency of the current program and in planning future marketing activities. What to measure can vary

Table 8.2 Northeast Multispecialty Group Referrals to Northside Hospital

Physician	*Jan*	*Feb*	*Mar*	*Apr*	*May*	*Jun*	*July*	*Total*
Bradley[a]	65	68	72	68	71	66	45	**455**
Smith[b]	15	14	20	18	28	30	35	**160**
Garcia[c]	160	140	132	156	149	152	138	**1027**
Chan[d]	0	0	23	20	28	32	48	**151**
Total	**240**	**222**	**247**	**262**	**276**	**280**	**266**	**1793**

[a]Based on the trend report, the marketing representative called on Dr. Bradley's office to find out why his referrals dipped in July. Was Dr. Bradley on vacation or was there a service problem that changed referrals?

[b]Marketing efforts for Dr. Smith concentrated on educating her about the expansion of services at the hospital, including DEXA scans and uterine fibroid embolization procedures. It is evident her referrals increased as she learned about the new procedures.

[c]Dr. Garcia has been consistent in his referrals to the facility. While he experienced service problems early in the year, they were promptly addressed and his patterns did not change. However, Dr. Garcia has a new office manager so the marketing staff has planned to increase visibility over the next few months until she is familiar with the imaging staff and services.

[d]Dr. Chan joined the group and rather than assume he would follow the referral patterns of his colleagues, the marketing representative spent time educating him about the equipment, services, radiologists, and insurance plans offered. His referrals increased consistently since that time.

from one year to the next or from one targeted marketing or advertising campaign to another. Evaluating individual elements of a marketing program can help identify those that are not working and need to be revised or eliminated. Given the difficulty in isolating the effects of any one marketing activity on healthcare customer behavior, however, the true value lies in a composite assessment.

Marketing results should also serve as a tool for operational management. Process lapses in carrying out procedures will negatively affect volume, revenue, and profitability. With their focus on meeting customers' needs and wants, marketing activities are often valuable communications mechanisms. Those responsible for collecting and analyzing marketing evaluation data can provide insights and

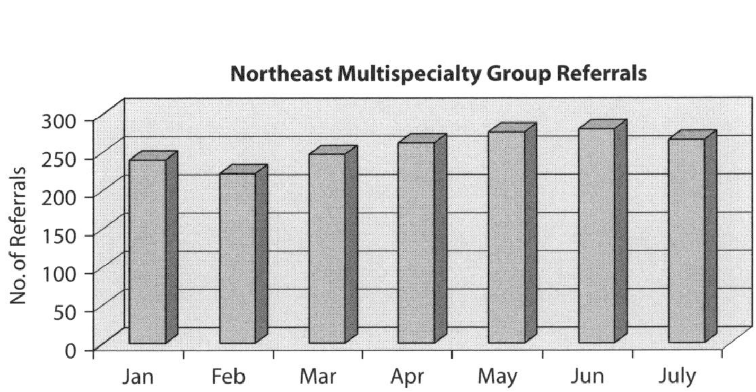

Figure 8.2 Northside Hospital Imaging Referral Totals

resources to prevent and resolve problems, which should be viewed as an important benefit of a marketing program.

References

1. Thomas RK. *Health Services Marketing: A Practitioner's Guide*. New York: Springer; 2008.
2. Hiebing RG Jr, Cooper SC. *The One-Day Marketing Plan*. 2nd ed. Lincolnwood, IL: NTC Business Books; 1999.

3 Customer Management and Satisfaction

In this section:

Chapter 9

Identify and Meet Customer Needs

Ernesto Cerdena

> *Customer service is at the core of sucessful business operations. The true delivery of the best service to customers is essential to survival. Not all customers are alike; each customer behaves differently based on his or her needs. Motivation is a theoretical concept that attempts to explain why people choose to engage in particular behaviors. It is essential for leaders to identify the needs of customers (patients and referring physicians) and promote a positive organizational culture in which employees are empowered to meet those needs. This, in turn, may lead to increased market share.*

An imaging facility must be focused in its aim to develop a proactive approach in identifying internal and external customer needs, specifically in regards to patients and referring physicians. With leadership driving the attention given to understanding the customer, service excellence can be realized by identifying the patient population, understanding their motivations and diverse backgrounds, and being sensitive and catering to wants and needs. Also, when organizational culture is aligned with performance, it empowers employees to provide excellent care and uphold the expected level of service.

Understanding Customer Motivation

Motivation and its associated concepts are often attributed to the variability of behavior, as they help explain the fact that under virtually identical external circumstances, there are great variations in individual behavior.[1] In addition, many experts argue that motivation is an inner drive that reflects goal-directed arousal. In a consumer behavior context, the desire for a product, service, or experience is the drive to satisfy needs and wants, both physiological and psychological, through the purchase and use of those products and services. Several theories, as well as the notion of diversity management and how it contributes to motivation, can aid in better understanding customer needs.

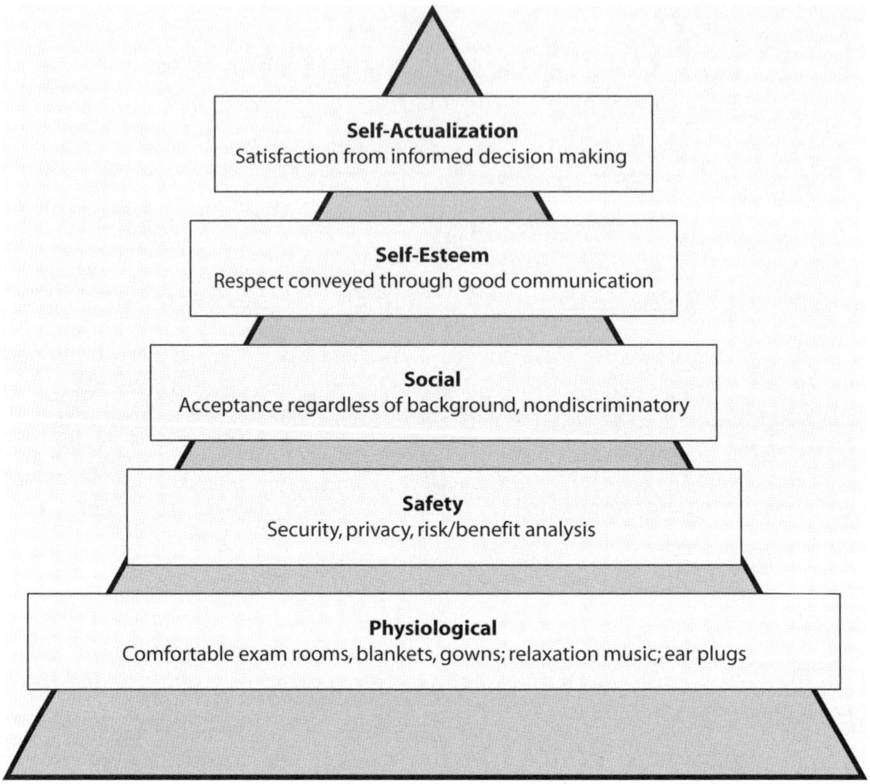

Figure 9.1 Maslow's Hierarchy of Needs Applied to an Imaging Facility

Motivational Theories

Motivation can be described as the process that accounts for an individual's intensity, direction, and persistent effort towards attaining a goal.[2] Understanding and identifying the customers' motivations are the means to exceed customer expectations. In medical imaging, patients and referring physicians have a choice and need to be given credible reasons to select and stay loyal to a facility.[3] Following are some basic theories of motivation.

Maslow's Hierarchy of Needs is one of the basic theories of motivation. Its simple, practical, and comprehensive approach is relevant to identifying customer needs in a diagnostic imaging facility. (Figure 9.1.) According to this theory, there is a hierarchy of five levels of human needs[4]:

1. *Physiological well-being.* This is the most basic of all human needs. It includes the need for food and shelter (or in the case of imaging, for example, comfortable exam rooms). An absence of these conditions is a big disincentive.
2. *Safety/Security.* People have the need to ensure that no personal harm will come to them. By meeting security, safety, and privacy needs, a facility may improve loyalty.

3. *Social validation.* This is the human need for acceptance by others, inclusion, friendship, and affection. Once the basic needs are met, customers will desire stimulating interaction with employees. They will want to feel important no matter what economic, generational, or ethnic background they come from. Some customers' motivations do not ever move past this level.
4. *Self-esteem.* This includes recognition, status, empowerment, and prestige. At this level, good communication, educational programs, and transparency are motivating factors.
5. *Self-actualization.* This is the need for achieving one's personal best. At this level, the driving force is completely internal. The customer is motivated and satisfied from creating and meeting challenges; empowerment, autonomy, and decision making serve the goal to prove that he made a difference. After a procedure, if the customer believes he made the right decision in choosing the service provider, he will be satisfied with the encounter and perhaps report this on any related survey.

Beyond this classic motivational theory, there are other theories that may help identify the needs of customers, such as the Fiedler contingency model, the Vroom-Yetton decision model, and the Hersey-Blanchard situational theory. In an organizational context, they emphasize the optimal course of action is contingent (dependent) upon the internal and external situation. Human behavior cannot be reduced to simple generalizations; but if one can identify enough characteristics of a situation—about prior experience of conditions, the human actors, properties of the task, and the environment within which the task is being carried out—one can then specify hypotheses or propositions.[5]

Diversity Management

Staff should display competency in dealing with customers regardless of age, ethnicity, religion, sexual orientation, and other such characteristics. Demographic variations and cultural backgrounds may cause customers to behave in certain ways and provide a basis for motivation when interacting with staff. Achieving excellent customer service means adhering to the core concepts of diversity management, a strategic and proactive process designed to develop and maintain a caring and inclusive workplace environment where differences are valued and integrated into an organization's day-to-day operations. This kind of exceptional workplace and business standard drives organizational high performance.[6]

Using generational cohorts as just one example, staff must work with customers of varying ages and understand the differing characteristics, attitudes, and life-shaping events that define them.[7] At this point in time, the customer base comprises four distinct generations each with its own values, expectations, and modes of communication[7]:

- People who lived during World War II. These are customers born between 1922 and 1943. They do not want to be rushed, and prefer a more relaxed pace that allows them to think through options and feel comfortable with outcomes. A rapport should be established with respect and in an "old-fashioned" way by addressing them as "sir" or "ma'am" and saying "please" and "thank you."
- Baby Boomers. These customers were born in the period 1943 to 1960. They value personalized treatment and have a strong sense of individuality, with many accustomed to being in the spotlight. Boomers prefer to be called by their first names and expect service that goes above and beyond to earn their loyalty.
- Generation X. Born between 1960 and 1980, this group is technologically savvy, clever, and resourceful. Customers from this generation expect efficient and to-the-point service. Competency is of the utmost importance.
- Generation Y, or Millenials. Born between 1980 and 2000, these customers are more sociable, optimistic, and practical. They are the first generation to grow up in the era of digital media. Despite being young, they expect respect and do not want to be spoken to with condescension.

Organizational Culture

The success of an imaging facility's efforts to deliver outstanding customer service rests on the organization's ability to recruit and retain top quality staff by creating and maintaining a culture built on principles of trust, inclusion, fairness, respect, and shared accountability. This focus on positive culture deliberately pursues a "performance culture" wherein anything that stands as a barrier to meeting or exceeding both clinical and workplace performance expectations is identified and promptly addressed.[6] Performance culture is built around a shared sense of commitment to exceeding expectations and achieving results relative to the organization's mission, vision, values, and objectives. Leadership is responsible for effectively aligning the objectives of every organizational process, system, and resource.

The most important management components of a successful customer experience are leadership engagement in taking ownership of the customer experience, followed by inclusion of key employees who are integral in linking the customers to the organization.[8] The successful implementation of outstanding customer service will not be realized without the full participation and support from the top leaders down to individuals who deal with customers. Customers expect value in addition to service. This value can be achieved through interdependent, positive working relationships of the entire team. Employees should aim to exceed the expectations of the customer by going above and beyond the call of duty. In performance oriented cultures, every effort is made to cultivate staff buy-in to this paradigm and participation with respect to decision making about the organization's, and each department's, strategic action plans. In this way, high performing staff seek and respond to opportunities to participate, continuously improve, and be held accountable for their work.[6]

Organizational leadership should empower frontline staff to resolve customer problems on their own. Proper orientation, training, and established policies and procedures provide employees with a solid foundation and creates a culture of consistency in which staff perform job expectations according to organizational standards. Additionally, the reenforcement of the organizational culture will help them perform with a positive and enthusiastic spirit. (Refer to AHRA's book *Human Resource Management in Radiology* for more on these topics.)

The first step in getting staff to go the extra mile and create loyal fans is to hire the right team with both competence and character.[9] Competency comes with people who have proven skills and experience in the job or people who have this potential; and character is found in people who share the vision and values of the organization. These are the employees who tend to bring an enormous understanding, passion, and enthusiasm to serving others.

There are three powerful reasons why employees are motivated to provide great customer service[10]:

1. Greater job satisfaction: Employees need to feel useful and productive; making a difference to the customer's experience allows them to take pride in their work. This sense of accomplishment increases job satisfaction and prevents job burnout.
2. Enhanced job success: Habitual delivery of the best quality service and techniques garners recognition from those who may be able to help an employee's career (eg, supervisors and managers). Using customer service skills effectively will make a great impression and can be considered as performance metrics toward a job promotion or merit increase.
3. Reduced stress: Learning to deliver quality customer service saves a lot of stress and hassle. Employees who practice these skills are routinely far less likely to experience protracted, unpleasant, and upsetting interactions with customers.

SIDEBAR 9.1: Five Rules for Setting and Meeting Expectations

- **Rule 1:** The patient is always right.
- **Rule 2:** If the patient is thought to be wrong, refer to Rule 1.
- **Rule 3:** Stay ahead of the curve.
- **Rule 4:** Remain flexibile.
- **Rule 5:** Utilize a persistent, low-key outreach.

Addressing the factors that contribute to developing a positive organizational culture (eg, focus on performance, leadership engagement, employee satisfaction and empowerment) will create positive perceptions about the staff and the organization, thus leading to better customer relationships.

Meeting Patient Needs

There are three basic needs that patients want to be met while in an imaging facility: access to service, minimal wait time, and quality of care. There are many ways to achieve the daunting and challenging tasks that solidify the profitability and stability of an organization, but keeping the core service strategy simple can be most effective. See Sidebar 9.1.

It is prudent for the staff to always be sensitive to and prepared to meet patient needs. According to a report conducted by Press Ganey, sensitivity to patient needs is one of the top listed priorities that require opportunities for improvements.[11] Sensitivity to patient needs begins with the attitude and knowledge of the scheduling personnel who help patients arrange immediate or convenient appointment times. Patients may be anxious about their medical conditions, in pain, or nervous about the results of their exams. They may also be suffering from financial distress due to lost time from work and medical bills. It is important for employees to demonstrate responsiveness to a high level of anxiety to ensure patients will have a positive experience.

Patients define good customer service not only by how much attention is given to them, but also by the profile of the imaging facility.[12] Most people form an impression in the first four seconds. This impression typically determines the tone and the tenor of the entirety of the relationship. The presentation of the department has a great influence on patient perception. It is imperative the waiting area is clean and in good order. Reading materials should be current and in wide variety that

Box 9.1 Patient Rights as the Customer

- **Problem resolution.** This is what customers want most. Even though employees cannot solve all problems, the team can create positive perceptions by addressing their concerns.
- **Effort.** Customers respect effort. They will turn if they sense their needs and wants are not being addressed.
- **Acknowledgement and understanding.** Customers expect their needs, wants, and concerns to be acknowledged and understood. They feel that active listening is a vital part of customer service.
- **Choice and options.** Customers want to feel that they are making the decisions and are being helped.
- **Positive surprises.** Customers appreciate the things that employees do to go above and beyond hopes and expectations.
- **Consistency, reliability, and predictability.** Customers expect the organization and its staff to deliver what was promised to them. By doing so, this creates customer loyalty.
- **Value.** Customers want the time and money they invest to equate to a superior quality service by experts.
- **Reasonable simplicity.** Customers do not want complicated processes—simple paperwork is most desirable.
- **Confidentiality.** Customers want and need full security for their personal information.
- **Sense of importance.** Customers want to be treated as partners.
- **Speed.** Prompt service is a customer priority.

Source: Adapted from Bacal R. *Perfect Phrases for Customer Service.* New York, New York: McGraw-Hill; 2005.

will match the interests of the patient demographic. Educational materials such as exam brochures may help ease fears. The front desk should be free from clutter and look neat and efficient. Staff should also be available to help patients complete specific exam questionnaires when requested. In addition, an insurance or patient access specialist should be available to assist patients in obtaining an authorization of the exam, thus reducing any additional stress that may be related to insurance concerns.

See Box 9.1 for a list of what patients want and need as the customer.

Access to Service

Access is a major component of the healthcare delivery system. Any impediment to diagnostic appointments may negatively impact patient care. Delays for appointments are prevalent, resulting in patient dissatisfaction, higher costs, and possible adverse clinical consequences.[13] To remedy this problem, many healthcare organizations identify a certain group of diagnostic services as "critical tests." This allows facilities to prioritize patients systematically and in a timely fashion. A strategic plan can also be developed that includes expansion of service hours with evenings and weekends; appointment time slots can also be adjusted to achieve full capacity, and blocks can be reserved for same-day add-ons and emergencies. When demands continue to increase, more equipment may be warranted in order to meet patient needs.

Wait Times

Excessive wait times in an imaging facility is a major dissatisfaction for patients, as they consider their time just as valuable as the staff's. As a result of excessive wait times, patients may judge their entire experience as negative. When it becomes unbearable, patients may resort to calling their primary care doctors and enlisting their help in getting to see referral specialists sooner.[14] This leads to a situation where a primary care doctor may feel pressured to exaggerate symptoms to obtain timely care for his patients.

An access problem such as this represents a delay between the initiation of the demand and the application of the supply. The goal in any system is to balance the demand with the supply. When this balance is achieved, wait times can be reduced or eliminated. Shorter wait times into specialty care improve patient satisfaction, physician satisfaction (on both the primary care and specialty sides), and staff satisfaction. Adverse clinical outcomes are averted, costs are reduced, and revenues are enhanced.[13]

Patient wait times can be identified in many ways depending upon the facility's protocols. Many organizations develop a color coding flag within the radiology information system (RIS) where the patient wait time can be tracked and quantified. For example, if the acceptable wait time is 10 minutes, all patients on the work list who are waiting for 10 minutes or more will change to a different color to alert the receptionists and technical staff. Some facilities may have a "customer service" advocate who effectively communicates about the wait time between the patients, support staff, and technical staff.

Reducing wait time can be managed through the elimination of inefficiencies in the workflow. Therefore, solid interdepartmental coordination should be consistently observed throughout the process, including test ordering, scheduling, exam preparations, reception, insurance authorization, technical staff, and test interpreting and reporting.

Quality of Care

Quality is a key indicator for customer service measurement and is another important dimension of meeting the needs of the patient. There are many areas that

SIDEBAR 9.2: The Planetree Model

Healthcare facilities in general continue to seek to improve their quality of care with particular attention to the patient experience. As one tool for survival, many are embracing the Planetree methodology, a patient-centric rather than provider-focused approach that helps improve quality outcomes in healthcare. The Planetree organization has been a pioneer in personalizing, humanizing, and demystifying the healthcare experience for patients and their families. It is committed to improving medical care from the patient's perspective and empowers people through information and education, encouraging "healing partnerships" with caregivers.

Planetree's approach is holistic and encourages healing in all dimensions—mental, emotional, spiritual and social, as well as physical. It seeks to maximize healthcare outcomes by integrating optimal medical therapies. Access to arts and nature are also incorporated into the healing environment. A study was conducted to link patient-centered care and quality outcomes, such as patient satisfaction. In this research, it was reported that the Planetree patient-centered model of care impacted the satisfaction of the healthcare team through an improved working environment. Hence, the delivery of quality of care was realized.

Sources: Planetree vision, mission and beliefs statements. Planetree, Inc. 2009. http://planetree.org/about.html. Accessed March 19, 2010.

Stone S. Planetree Implementation Improves Quality Outcomes. Plane*talk*. October 2007. Available at: http://planetree.org/Planetalk_October_2007_Susan_Stone.pdf. Accessed March 19, 2010.

customers are paying attention to, including report turnaround time, image quality, appropriateness of the test, and overall interaction with the staff. See Sidebar 9.2 for a specific methodology for improving quality of care.

Improvements in the quality of care depend on the organization's ability to elicit and monitor customer complaints. In particular, service recovery cannot take place if the organization does not know that the customer is unhappy. Many people would rather "switch than fight," especially in a healthcare environment, where people fear that complaining could jeopardize the quality of the clinical care they receive. Also, minorities and people from underserved communities tend to avoid complaining, even though they may have significant problems with the delivery of care.[15,16] See Table 9.1.

Meeting Referring Physician Needs

It is paramount to cultivate relationships with referring physicians in order to meet their needs. A facility can enter into a strategic partnership with a referring physician to ensure patients aren't sent to competitors. Once the alliance has been established,

Table 9.1 How to Use Complaint Management as an Effective Service Recovery Tool

Complaint Management Process Step	*Actions to Take*
1. Encourage use of complaints as a QI tool.	■ Let staff know that complaints are valued and essential for QI. ■ Display complaints in public areas to reinforce the value you place on them. ■ Make it easy for customers and staff to complain.
2. Establish a team of people to respond to complaints.	■ Include in the team people from the front lines as well as senior management. ■ Use this team to develop planned protocols for service recovery for the most common service failures.
3. Resolve customer problems quickly and effectively.	■ Commit the organization to resolving complaints quickly to avoid the waste of repeated contacts. ■ Train and empower frontline employees to resolve problems and give them the authority to fix problems on the spot.
4. Develop a complaint database.	■ Develop a computerized database that catalogs complaints by CAHPS composite or question. ■ Use the database to identify trends and generate regular reports to staff and management.
5. Commit to identifying failure points in the system.	■ Using complaint data, identify failure points that are root causes of low satisfaction. ■ Be proactive, not reactive; try to anticipate negative situations from occurring in the first place.
6. Track trends and use information to improve service processes.	■ Stop handling problems one at a time as if they have never occurred before.

QI, quality improvement; CAHPS, Consumer Assessment of Healthcare Providers and Systems

Source: Adapted from Bendall-Lyon D, Powers TL. The role of complaint management in the service recovery process. *Jt Comm J Qual Improv.* 2001 May;27(5):278–86.

it is important to maintain the relationship by regular communications between the offices to keep abreast of any problems that may cause a loss of referrals. Also, any patient-related issues and concerns should be proactively communicated to the referring physician.

Common issues that arise from referring physicians and their office staff revolve around scheduling, report turnaround, and access to images. Attention to these concerns not only allows a facility to meet referring physician expectations, but contributes significantly to the delivery of quality patient care.

Scheduling

Most referring physicians rely on office staff when deciding where to schedule their patients for diagnostic imaging studies. If the staff has difficulty connecting to one facility, it is likely the patient will be scheduled to a different imaging facility. The scheduling system should be simple and quick. Exam prep materials should be easily accessible online or by fax. And importantly, the friendliness, courtesy, helpfulness, efficiency, and professionalism of the scheduling staff are absolutely necessary to make the process effective and successful.

Report Turnaround

If an imaging facility promises to have a certain report turnaround time, then it must deliver it. Referring physicians do not want to deal with excuses for the delay of reports. The only acceptable cause of a delay is the need to compare studies with outside films. A stat reading request for reports must be honored as soon possible by a direct phone call from the radiologist to the ordering physician—especially if the results are critical. The imaging facility should establish a simple, user-friendly system for the report to be easily accessible to the referring physician. This could be sent via e-mail (encrypted), fax, or mail. It is important to have a back-up mechanism should one system fail.

Access to Images

With the advent of filmless technology, accessibility to diagnostic images has become easier. An imaging facility may elect to set up an individual account for key referring physicians to access the imaging facility's PACS or imaging database through the installation of a virtual private network (VPN). Observing the HIPAA regulations when establishing this connection is an important consideration. Another option is providing patients with copies of the completed studies on CDs or DVDs so the patients will have copies for their records and to provide to their referring physicians.

Conclusion

Meeting the needs of customers is an essential part of providing quality service. This can be realized by identifying the patient and physician population, understanding their motivations, and being sensitive and catering to specific wants and needs. Establishing and cultivating relationships with referring physicians and their staff also promotes a stable workload. Moreover, the organizational culture should be aligned with performance, which will allow employees to uphold the expected level of service. In line with the mission and vision of the organization, a creative and innovative customer service program can be established. Once in place, the entire organizational structure, from administration to support staff, should work together to successfully deliver the whole customer service package to patients and their families, as well as referring physicians and their office staff.

References

1. Beck RC. *Motivation: Theories and Principles*. Upper Saddle River, NJ: Prentice-Hall; 2000:2–3.
2. Robbins S, Judge T. *Organizational Behavior*. Upper Saddle River, NJ: Prentice-Hall; 2007:186.
3. Zahaluk D. Patient retention strategies—impression management. Available at: http://ezinearticles.com/?Patient-Retention-Strategies---Impression-Management&id=1877658. Accessed January 18, 2009.
4. Archer LH, Lewis R, Spearing S (eds). *Human Resource Management in Radiology*. Sudbury, MA: AHRA; 2008.
5. Schein E. *Organizational Psychology*. Upper Saddle River, NJ: Prentice-Hall; 1980:48–49.
6. Strelitz P, Watson K. Achieving high performance through organizational culture transformation: key concepts and best practices, part 1. *Radiol Manage*. 2009;31(3):28–33.
7. Performance Research Associates. *Delivering Knock Your Socks Off Service*. New York, NY: American Management Association; 2007:103–108.
8. Lutz S, Foong S. A strategy fit for a king: a customer experience framework. American College of Healthcare Executives: *J Healthcare Manage*. November/December 2008;53(6):356–357.
9. Blanchard K. *Customer Mania! It's Never too Late to Build Customer-Focused Company*. New York, NY: Free Press; 2004:74–75.
10. Bacal R. *Perfect Phrases for Customer Service*. New York, NY: McGraw-Hill; 2005:3–12.
11. Clark PA. Medical practices' sensitivity to patients' needs: opportunities and practice improvement. *J Ambulatory Care Manage*: April/June 2003;26(2):110–123.
12. Kroken P. At your service: how do your customers feel. *Radiol Manage*. 2006. Available at: http://www.ahraonline.org/RM/RMShow.asp?ID=637. Accessed April 25, 2007.
13. Green LV, Savin S, Murray M. Providing timely access to care: what is the right patient panel size? *The Joint Commission Journal on Quality and Patient Safety*. 2007;33(4):211–218.

14. Murray M. Reducing waits and delays in the referral process. American Academy of Family Physicians' Family Practice Management. 2002; March. Available at: http://www.aafp.org/fpm/20020300/39redu.html. Accessed January 18, 2009.

15. Schneider EC, Zaslavsky AM, Landon BE, Lied TR, Sheingold S, Cleary PD. National quality monitoring of Medicare health plans: the relationship between enrollees' reports and the quality of clinical care. Med Care 2001;39(12):1313–1325.

16. Zaslavsky AM, Zaborski LB, Cleary PD. Factors affecting response rates to the Consumer Assessment of Health Plans Study survey. Med Care 2002;40(6):485–499.

Chapter 10

Commit to Measuring Satisfaction

Kathy Tabor McEwan and Barbara Hubley

The ability to "prove" customer satisfaction by quantified measurement has become increasingly important to the individual consumer, government and accrediting agencies, employers, referring physicians, and third-party payers. Measuring patient and physician satisfaction meets the demands of these individuals and organizations and also contributes to the facility's bottom line, market share, continuous quality improvement efforts, market strategy, and organizational planning.

As the business of healthcare has matured, preparing accurate budgets, controlling costs, effectively competing, and establishing a sound market position have become top priorities. The bottom line and return on investment must be continually analyzed and facilities must strategize about what it will take to survive and get ahead. Healthcare facilities are being scrutinized by accrediting agencies, government regulators, third-party payers, patients, referring physicians, and communities. Among the elements under the microscope is the quality of the services provided.

While quantifying satisfaction presents challenges, the reasons to measure it far outweigh the difficulties. An organization that is unable or unwilling to maintain or improve satisfaction will not survive in the future.[1] See also Sidebar 10.1 for key points on why measuring satisfaction is relevant.

Retaining customers and building market share have a positive impact on a facility's bottom line and can contribute to cost efficiencies. Measuring satisfaction and using it to guide quality improvements appear to affect a facility's financial success in other ways. A study of Veterans Administration ambulatory care centers found that facilities with higher patient-perceived service quality and patient satisfaction had lower average treatment costs.[2]

Measuring customer satisfaction matters. Knowing why it matters to a specific facility and using that knowledge to establish goals for measuring the facility's

SIDEBAR 10.1: Why Measure Satisfaction?

- To understand what the customer wants
- To better respond to customers
- To gather information needed to define superior service and establish a service strategy
- To set standards and measure performance
- To empower employees to work for the customer
- To recognize and reward accomplishment

customer satisfaction levels comprise the first step in creating an effective program to ensure quality customer service (Figure 10.1).

Patient Satisfaction

Researchers postulate that patients make evaluations based on a subjective standard. As the patient's valuation shifts toward the standard, the result is satisfaction. As the variance between the standard and the valuation increases, so does the likelihood of dissatisfaction. Patients make judgments on the aspects of quality they are capable of appreciating.[1] Patient satisfaction is one of 26 criteria that have been used to define quality of care from the patient's perspective.[3] The patient's expectations determine the quality standards. Quality judgments are the result of the patient's perception of service level minus his or her expectation of what the level would be.

The patient's evaluation of quality incorporates both a cognitive evaluation and an emotional reaction that can challenge any attempts to measure satisfaction.

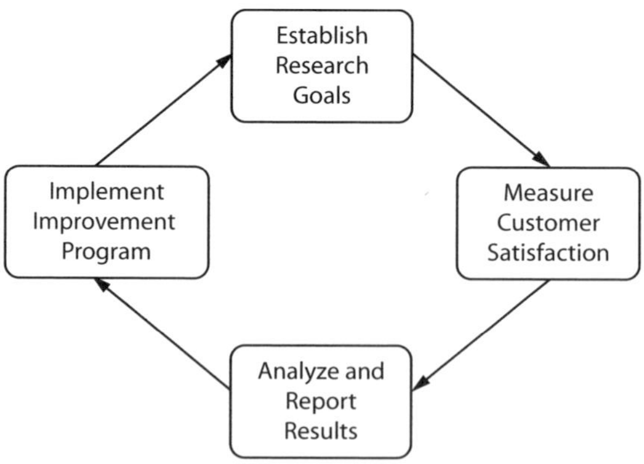

Figure 10.1 Customer Satisfaction Cycle

With Internet access and health-focused print and television programming, it has never been easier for patients and families to gather information and statistics related to their healthcare and to providers. This increases the likelihood that the patient's cognitive evaluation will be based on valid information. It also increases the patient's expectations, sometimes to an unrealistic level (eg, patients expect hospitals, regardless of size, to have the latest technologically advanced equipment, while financial constraints may prohibit leasing or purchasing such equipment).

Increasingly, patients are insisting on having a say in where they will receive care. Satisfaction has been shown to correlate with the amount of choice the patient had in the purchasing decision.[4] For example, patients whose employers give them a choice of healthcare plans have been found to give higher ratings on provider satisfaction surveys than do those who had no choice. This leaves providers to wonder just how much control they have over the results of any satisfaction survey.

Accrediting agencies, third-party payers, and corporate owners are among the external drivers pushing healthcare organizations to continually measure patient satisfaction. Both The Joint Commission and the National Committee on Quality Assurance have quality indicators that include patient satisfaction. Nearly one-third of the points needed to achieve the Malcolm Baldrige National Quality Award relate to customer satisfaction criteria, including complaint resolution and service standards.

The cost to acquire a new customer may be up to five times that of retaining an existing one.[5] Dissatisfied and unhappy customers can be costly in other ways, in particular, by discouraging others from using the service. Some research has shown a connection between customer satisfaction and loyalty as indicated by declaring the intention of using a service provider again.[2] Other factors (such as a change of insurer) may intervene to prevent declared behavioral intentions from consistently predicting actual behavior. Customer loyalty seems to be linked with the customer's assessment of the organization's reliability (as demonstrated by its ability to perform the service accurately and dependably) and assurance (as conveyed by its staff's ability to engender trust and confidence and exhibit courtesy).[6]

An organization may not fully understand what its customers want unless it is willing to measure it. In addition to assessing the organization's reliability and assurance, patients consider responsiveness (willingness to help and provide prompt service), empathy (caring, individualized attention), and tangibles (physical facilities, equipment, and staff appearance). Healthcare administrators, employees, and physicians consistently overestimate the patients' expectations for tangibles and underestimate their expectations for the other features.[7] Measuring satisfaction is one tool that can be used to more accurately assess what matters to patients and better meet those expectations.

Physician Satisfaction

While the core focus of most organizations tends to be on measuring the satisfaction of patients, it is also important to analyze that of referring physicians whose referrals provide an external impetus to measure (and manage) overall satisfaction. Oftentimes, it is the referring physician's office who can influence volume in deciding where their patients will receive imaging services. So the ability to "prove" customer satisfaction has become increasingly important to multiple parties.

Being able to anticipate problems and take action to prevent their occurrence are key characteristics of service-oriented organizations and are invaluable in building and maintaining market share. As well as patient satisfaction data, physician satisfaction data can be instrumental in highlighting service failures. Organizations that can resolve these issues are also more likely to retain them as customers.

Links to Employee Satisfaction

Satisfied employees provide quality patient care, which leads to patient satisfaction.[8] Employee perceptions of customer service are linked to customer perceptions of high-quality service.[2] In particular, employees who work in a high-performance work environment and are focused on employee involvement, empowerment, goal alignment, training, teamwork, and performance-based awards feel they are able to deliver high-quality patient service. In turn, the patients they serve perceive the service to be high-quality and express high levels of satisfaction.

Good interactions between service providers and customers often result in customer satisfaction despite any deficiencies with other aspects of service delivery. If a customer experiences dissatisfaction with one aspect of service delivery it could result in dissatisfaction with other aspects that would have otherwise been pleasant.[9] Administrators who make large attempts to improve employee satisfaction are more successful at improving customer satisfaction and improved customer satisfaction leads to a larger volume of customers.[10]

Employee satisfaction is covered in depth in AHRA's book *Human Resource Management in Radiology*.

Conclusion

Typically, what gets measured gets managed.[1] Data from satisfaction measurements can help administrators identify areas that need improvement, plan new services, revise existing services, and develop employee training programs. These data help managers focus on what went wrong, rather than on who is at fault. Satisfaction data can provide the basis for the facility's continuing quality improvement efforts and guide marketing strategy.

Satisfaction is measured because it is critical to understand the customer and respond to their needs. An organization should have a management team committed to and focused on its customers by:

- Knowing what customers want and meeting those needs
- Knowing and publishing its performance measurements, including patient satisfaction data
- Implementing systems and strategies based on past performance measures and thus are customer friendly
- Training and empowering its employees to care for customers
- Rewarding and recognizing improvements

If a facility cannot or will not supply data on satisfaction rates, customers may choose to look elsewhere for the information and ultimately for service. Meeting these standards will create a positive image, retain customers, increase revenue, decrease waste, breed motivated staff, and grow repeat business and market share.

References

1. Ford RC, Bach SA, Fottler MD. Methods of measuring patient satisfaction in health care organizations. *Health Care Manage Rev.* 1997;22(2):74–89.

2. Scotti DJ, Harmon J, Behson SJ. Links among high-performance work environment, service quality, and customer satisfaction: an extension to the healthcare sector. *J Healthc Manag.* 2007;52:109–124.

3. van Campen C, Sixma H, Friele RD, Kerssens JJ, Peters L. Quality of care and patient satisfaction: a review of measuring instruments. *Med Care Res Rev.* 1995;52:109–133.

4. Ullman R, Hill JW, Scheye EC, Spoeri RK. Satisfaction and choice: a view from the plans. *Health Aff (Millwood).* 1997;16:209–217.

5. Clarke RN. Marketing healthcare services. In: Wolper LF. *Health Care Administration: Planning, Implementing, and Managing Organized Delivery Systems*. 4th ed. Boston, MA: Jones and Bartlett; 2004: 435.

6. Griffith JR, White KR. *The Well-Managed Healthcare Organization*. 5th ed. Chicago, IL: AUPHA Press; 2002:191.

7. O'Connor SJ, Trinh HQ, Shewchuk RM. Perceptual gaps in understanding patient expectations for health care service quality. *Health Care Manage Rev*. 2000;25(2):7–23.

8. Jackson T, Wood B. Employee and customer satisfaction in healthcare. *Radiology Management*. 2010;32(2):20–25.

9. Brown SP, Lam SK. A meta-analysis of relationships linking employee satisfaction to customer responses. *Journal of Retailing*. 2008;84(3):243–255.

10. Zondiros Z, Konstantoplous N, Tomaras P. A simulation model for measuring customer satisfaction through employee satisfaction. *Computation in Modern Science and Engineering*. 2008;2:1086–1089.

Chapter 11

Measure Satisfaction: Qualitative and Quantitative Tools

Kathy Tabor McEwan and Barbara Hubley

Customer satisfaction is one indicator of quality healthcare. There is a range of tools that can be used to collect and analyze qualitative and quantitative data on a facility's satisfaction levels. The category of customer (eg, referring physicians or patients), the information's ultimate use, available expertise, and the facility's time line and budget determine the method to use.

Given the importance of measuring customer satisfaction to healthcare organizations, it is perhaps not surprising that considerable time, money, and effort are spent on evaluating and selecting the right approach to measurement. Used properly, the data gathered will guide continuous quality improvement efforts, employee development, procedural changes, implementation of new or revised services, and more. "Selecting the best method or combination of methods should represent an ideal balance between the organization's strategic goals and the cost of achieving those goals."[1] Thus, it is important that the findings from measuring customer satisfaction be accurate and appropriate for the intended use.

General Considerations in Method Selection

Satisfaction measurement methods follow one of two general approaches. Qualitative methodology collects detailed customer feedback through such means as focus groups and managerial observation. It offers insights into customers' responses to both the service received and their experience with it. Quantitative methodology relies on standardized questions such as surveys. Its results lend themselves to mathematical analysis and tend to be more accurate than those of qualitative measures. As will be discussed later, all the tools used in these methods vary in accuracy of findings, timeliness of information gathered, cost to implement, and convenience to respondents.

Sequencing inquiries into different areas of patient satisfaction also determines approach. For example, if there is an issue with the registration process, it might be beneficial to conduct either a focus group with a handful of patients or one-on-one management interviews. Doing this prior to developing a larger, quantitative patient satisfaction survey will aid in designing the best possible survey tool. Or, conversely, if comments collected from a broadly administered quantitative survey suggest there is a problem with patient wait times, it may be worthwhile to drill down into the issue. Among the analytical options are conducting a detailed follow-up quantitative survey focusing only on wait times that breaks down all possible causes of patients waiting, or reaching out to patients who are waiting through one-on-one interviews.

Other considerations that enter into selecting a tool are its potential for bias, validity, reliability, and generalizability, as well as timing.

Potential for Bias

All satisfaction measurement methods may produce biased results that can affect the accuracy and usefulness of the data. Among the possible sources of bias are[1]:

1. Nonresponse bias: Nonrespondents hold a less favorable view of their experience than respondents.
2. Mode of administration bias: Personal interviews tend to result in not only higher response rates, but also higher levels of satisfaction.
3. Timing bias: Customers surveyed within a few days or weeks of their service tend to express lower levels of satisfaction than those surveyed at the time of service or several months later.
4. Response format bias: Questions that are open ended or use multiple response scales (eg, a Likert 5-point scale) tend to draw lower levels of satisfaction than close-ended questions or those using a 2-point scale.
5. Proxy bias: A patient's relative or proxy may rank service more negatively than does the patient.
6. End-user bias: Interpretation of resulting data can be subjective.

Among the best ways to prevent bias and increase the likelihood of accurate responses are to use multiple formats and vary the timing. For other suggestions of ways to enhance results, see Sidebar 11.1.

Validity, Reliability, and Generalizability

Failure to establish validity or reliability oftentimes happens when individuals create their own satisfaction tools. In an analysis of 131 instruments to measure quality of care from the patient's perspective, only 41 had been tested even once for

SIDEBAR 11.1: Guidelines for Measuring Customer Satisfaction

- Use multiple sources of satisfaction data.
- Get management and employee commitment.
- Involve customers in the tool development process.
- Make sure the information collected is both important to the respondent and useful for management decision making.
- Decide whether data will be gathered for all customers of a specific category (eg, patients, referring physicians) or just a sample.
- If sampling, make sure the sample is representative.
- Use existing instruments as a starting point rather than creating one from scratch whenever possible.
- For surveys, pretest questions to ensure clarity and accuracy of response.
- Validate responses by gathering data on a given sample for more than one time period.
- Collect data within 1 week (interviews) or 1 month (questionnaires) of the respondent's service encounter.
- Order the questions to follow the sequence of the respondent's service encounter.
- Use both open-ended and closed-ended questions.
- Offer more than two possible responses.

Source: Adapted from Ford RC, Bach SA, Fottler MD. Methods of measuring patient satisfaction in health care organizations. *Health Care Manage Rev*. 1997;22(2):74-89.

reliability or validity.[2] Reliability relates to the consistency of results from one use of an instrument to another, and validity refers to the accuracy with which the instrument actually measures what is sought. Techniques that are both reliable and valid will produce dependable data that can be used to guide strategic goals and can be compared over time to demonstrate improvement. In addition, validity influences generalizability, the application of the data across a wide population, an important consideration for large, multisystem organizations with a diverse patient population.

Reliability is improved when questions are clearly and carefully crafted and the instrument contains numerous questions, and can be evaluated by giving it twice and applying a correlation coefficient. For improved validity, the tool should be used with the largest reasonable sample size because the larger the sample, the greater the validity (see Sidebar 11.2). The simplest way to ensure reliability, validity, and generalizability is to start with an existing, well-tested instrument and make minor adjustments, if necessary, to meet the needs of the facility.[2]

Timing

As noted previously, the timing of a measurement process can introduce bias into the results by affecting the customer's expressed level of satisfaction. In addition, the

SIDEBAR 11.2: Sampling Vocabulary

Sample frame—the entire customer base or customers in one or more categories of the base (eg, referring physicians). The difficulty often comes in defining just who is the customer. In the case of referring physicians, for example, does the frame include their staff members who schedule tests? Does it include only physicians who have referred a patient within the past year?

Census—research based on the entire sample frame; only if the frame is relatively small does a census make sense financially to most facilities.

Sample—research based on a representative selection from the sample frame. There are two different methods of selecting samples. *Probability* sampling uses a random system of selecting participants that ensures each has an equal chance to end up in the sample (eg, every fifth name). This method of sampling allows the researcher to calculate the exact size of sample needed (and thereby the cost of the research), select a usefully representative cross-section of clients, and know the margin of error. *Nonprobability* samples are selected based on criteria determined by the research goals; the sample is targeted to specifics such as a quota (eg, 25 men and 25 women) or a demographic. Qualitative tools can be used with nonprobability sampling when the sample size is small and the goal is not to generalize the results from the survey group to the entire population.

Among the useful resources for more information about sampling methods are:

McQuarrie EF. *Market Research Toolbox: A Concise Guide for Beginners*. 2nd ed. Thousand Oaks, CA: Sage Publications; 2006.

Naumann E, Giel K. *Customer Satisfaction Measurement and Management*. Milwaukee, WI: ASQ Quality Press; 1995.

Scheaffer RL, Mendenhall W, Ott RL. *Elementary Survey Sampling*. 6th ed. Florence, KY: Cengage Learning; 2005.

longer the time interval between the service and the survey, the less likely the customer is to respond. Measuring customer satisfaction at the time of service, when possible, has the added advantage of allowing correction of any problems before the customer leaves the facility. If satisfaction cannot be measured at the time of service, it is generally advisable to do so within 1–4 weeks.

Qualitative Tools to Measure Satisfaction

Qualitative measures are particularly useful to identify what matters most to customers, whether there are any unmet needs or preferred features, and how a facility's services compare with its competitors. These tools are often used to identify the attributes to be subsequently measured by quantitative tools. While focus groups are probably the most popular qualitative methodology used in healthcare, others may be useful in certain settings, including managerial observations and employee feedback.

Focus Groups

Focus groups have historically been a common tool in market research, but have become more widely used in healthcare as a way to gather qualitative data for needs assessment, outcome evaluation, program improvements, and organizational development.[3] Focus groups can also be an effective tool to determine what service elements and attributes are important to patients.[1]

Focus groups involve gathering seven to ten people together to discuss a specific topic, guided by a trained facilitator. A defining characteristic is the interaction among group members, often leading to members recalling additional experiences and feelings and developing viewpoints during the session. This interaction is encouraged by the open-ended questions used to guide discussion. A group session will last from 60 minutes to several hours, depending on the topic to be discussed, the budget, and the availability of participants. Conducting several sessions with different participants each time will increase the validity of the data collected. The following should be kept in mind to ensure the best results from a focus group[4]:

- Clearly identify the purpose of the focus group and what information is sought.
- Select participants based on the research topic (eg, patients who have undergone mammography if the organization is considering expanding its mammography services).
- Select an environment that is conducive to conversation.
- Use an exercise or material such as film clips or cartoons to break the ice and stimulate discussion.
- Use short, natural, open-ended questions.
- Have information (eg, facility brochures) available, should participant questions arise about services.
- Make sure the facilitator has appropriate contact names and numbers that can be given to a participant who reveals a sensitive issue that should be dealt with by a physician or other professional.

Focus groups are particularly valuable in gathering information on (1) customers' views of the facility's services; (2) the reasons participants think the way they do about the facility; and (3) directions to take for adding or revising services.

The process can be used with referring physicians and their staffs to evaluate physician services as well as with patients and/or their families to evaluate patient services.

When compared with most quantitative instruments, focus groups are a relatively inexpensive tool. Depending on the participants, a group can be assembled fairly quickly and the responses are immediate. The discussion can reveal issues previously unrecognized by the organization and draw out rich details that can provide direction to subsequent quantitative measures. Research indicates that focus groups can be effective in accessing views of members of traditionally hard to reach groups (eg, ethnic minority women).[4]

On the other hand, focus groups produce large volumes of qualitative data that must be precisely transcribed and then analyzed. The data are highly context specific, so extrapolating conclusions must be done very carefully. For example, if comments are taken out of context and used to assign priorities for service funding, the results may not be as expected.[4] Focus group costs can be more than anticipated, especially as more than one session will usually be needed, and can include: rental of a suitable meeting space; hiring a trained facilitator and transcriber and paying their expenses; staff time to identify and contact participants, follow up to ensure attendance, and make arrangements; compensatory stipends to participants; refreshments; and data analysis. Other disadvantages include the lack of anonymity for participants, the potential that one or more participants will dominate the discussion, and the lack of generalizability for the results because participants are essentially self-selected and not necessarily a representative sampling.

Online focus groups

As Internet access has broadened, conducting focus groups online has become a viable option for healthcare research. Terminology varies (eg, electronic focus groups, virtual panel discussions), but the key features are a text-based group discussion on a specific topic, guided by a moderator. These are not chat rooms or open panel discussions that allow participants to log in at any time and post comments on a random subject.[5]

Online focus groups can be set up using courseware designed to build Web-based learning environments. Participants do not need special software, only an Internet connection. The group can be conducted synchronously, asynchronously, or a combination of both. A synchronous group is conducted in real time, with all participants logging in at a predetermined time, receiving postings, and immediately responding. Asynchronous groups, on the other hand, allow participants to log in at a time that suits them within a specified time frame, read other participants' comments, and then post their own comments.

A key advantage of online focus groups is also one of its fundamental disadvantages. Experience shows that the format is able to attract participants who have been hard to reach with traditional focus groups (eg, disabled, socially isolated, young people).[5] At the same time, the format may dissuade from actively participating those who are not computer literate, who do not have easy Internet access, or for whom English (or the primary language of the group) is a second language.

Other advantages include[5,6]:

- The flexibility participants have to log in and post comments, increasing the likelihood of taking part
- The reduction in costs related to moderator travel, venue, refreshments, etc.
- The ease with which relatively large groups can be moderated by a single person
- The automatic and accurate capture of discussion data, eliminating the need for transcription
- Potential anonymity by using software that allows each participant to log in using a unique username and password
- Greater equality of participation than with traditional focus groups because one participant is unable to intimidate others or control the discussion
- Responses that tend to be lengthier and more considered than in traditional groups, enhancing the accuracy and objectivity of the data

The technology of the online format also introduces distinctive disadvantages over face-to-face groups, including[7]:

- The lack of nonverbal cues
- Respondents' written communication skills introduce potential for misinterpretations
- The moderator is unable to verify that the person logging in and commenting is in fact the person who is registered to do so
- Problems with software compatibility and file conversions, especially if a survey has international participants, can introduce unpredictable issues that may interfere with participation and bias the results
- Privacy and confidentiality cannot be assured—no online interaction is completely secure, nor are data completely safe from intrusion

To make the most of an online focus group, straightforward questions should be designed, introducing each over a period of time (eg, one per day), rather than all at once. The participants should be given a specified time period within which to respond, with a reminder or reminders, if necessary. The survey should have a defined end point. Because of the technical issues, it is advisable to involve a computer technician in the set-up and design and to monitor problems as they arise. All participants should be informed about how their messages will be used and that the possibility for interception exists. If a username and password are used, participants should be reminded about the need for keeping them safe to protect everyone in the group.

Managerial Observations

Managers often informally observe interactions between staff and customers, but a more formal program of managerial monitoring can be a low-cost way of gathering qualitative data. Anyone who has called an organization and listened to a recording announcing that "this call may be monitored for training and quality assurance purposes" has experienced one form of managerial observation. Whether in person or via recording, such observations take advantage of the manager's knowledge of the organization, its staff, and its policies and procedures. The method is probably one of the least expensive and simplest measurement tools to implement. It involves little, if any, inconvenience to the customer. Perhaps most importantly, should the manager observe a service problem, he or she can intervene to "course correct."

Relying on managers to observe employees, of course, introduces the possibility of personal bias or of misinterpretation. Since a manager cannot observe every patient or referring physician interaction, the sample will be small. Nor is it necessarily representative of every encounter, because when a manager is observing, it may influence how employees perform their jobs.

Managerial observation is more likely to provide useful data if the following guidelines are followed[1]:

1. Managers should be trained in structured observation techniques.
2. Managers should be familiar with the patient demographics and clinical processes to be observed.
3. Observations should focus on elements important to patients and on quality standards for which employees are responsible.
4. Observations can be made randomly, unobtrusively, or via video camera to lessen the effect on employee behavior. However, employees should be told they are subject to monitoring.
5. Observations should be made over various time periods.

Employee Feedback

If quality problems are traced back to their root causes, about 85% of the time the organization's system, processes, practices, and structure are at fault; an employee who was not conscientious or did not care is at fault only about 15% of the time.[1] Using employee feedback can highlight many of these system failures and suggestions of ways to correct them, which will have a positive impact on customer satisfaction. Employees base their comments on their own observations and experiences with customers, as well as on customer comments about problems "with the system."

Feedback programs tend to be episodic and may rely on some form of "incident report" with follow-up. A manager may empower employees to take action immediately to correct designated types of customer problems with an after-the-fact report and recommendations for permanent changes. In such cases, recovery from the service failure can be immediate and customer loyalty retained (service recovery should also be proportional to the problem). Feedback programs also have the advantages of being inexpensive and easy to implement. There is no inconvenience to patients, and employee morale is heightened by empowerment.

Just Culture

The goal of a "just culture" is to achieve an organizational environment in which frontline personnel feel comfortable disclosing errors—including their own—while maintaining professional accountability. It's about:

- Creating an open, fair, and just culture
- Developing a learning culture
- Designing safe systems
- Managing behavioral choices

Traditionally, healthcare's culture has held individuals accountable for errors or mishaps that befall patients under their care. By contrast, a just culture recognizes that individuals should not be held accountable for system failings over which they have no control. A just culture also recognizes many errors represent predictable interactions between people and the systems in which they work. However, in contrast to a culture that touts "no blame" as its governing principle, a just culture does not tolerate conscious disregard of clear risks to patients or gross misconduct (eg, falsifying a record, performing professional duties while intoxicated).[8]

Though an organization can't guarantee perfect outcomes, it "can commit to maximizing its reliability around each of its core values and being the best steward of the limited resources it has."[9]

Quality Circles

Quality circles serve to empower employees. While they elicit some of the same types of information as employee feedback programs, the circles involve continuous employee input through a team approach. They are formal groups comprised of employees in similar job classifications who volunteer to meet regularly—at least once a week—during the workday. Depending on the organization's size, the circle may have eight to ten members. They are trained in the basics of problem identification, information gathering and analysis, and solution generation. The focus of their efforts varies with the facility but tends to be process improvements, workplace issues, and other quality issues that affect performance and customer satisfaction. The group presents its recommendations to management and may be asked to conduct a follow-up analysis if those recommendations are implemented.

An effective quality circle builds employee morale through empowerment and efficiency through teamwork. Customers are better served because team members tend to strive consistently for quality, while conveying confidence and competence. Because circles meet regularly to deal with a variety of issues, rather than being an ad hoc solution to a single problem, the organization benefits from the continuity and from the knowledge gained by the participants over time. On the other hand, quality circles only work when management trusts its employees enough to fully empower them and when employees can work together as a cohesive team in a "no-fault" environment. Management must also be willing to accommodate the considerable time commitment involved.

Table 11.1 summarizes the features of qualitative measurement tools.

Quantitative Tools to Measure Satisfaction

The most direct method of gathering information from any customer is to conduct a survey. Simply following a hunch or making assumptions about how well the organization is responding to constituent needs is not enough in today's competitive, monitored healthcare environment. The quantitative responses from a survey can be the starting point for operational improvements that enhance the customer experience. For example, survey results can:

- Identify a recurring problem or similarity in the surveyed population (eg, key words can be searched and selected)
- Give the organization top items to focus on and rank them in order of importance
- Allow for benchmarking against peer groups and trend analysis

Table 11.1 Features of Qualitative Measurement Tools

Tool	*Cost Factors*	*Time line*	*Confidentiality*	*Risks*
Managerial observation	Low	Immediate	Not achieved	Lacks validity and reliability Specialized training needed Employee behavior influenced by observation
Employee feedback	Low	Immediate; if using written reports, 1–3 days	Not achieved	Specialized training needed Lacks validity and reliability
Quality circle	Cost relatively high because of considerable staff time needed	Ongoing	Customer, but not staff, confidentiality may be achieved	Specialized training needed Cohesive team needed Staff capable of using empowerment
Focus group	Tends to be costly	Immediate for participants; 1–4 weeks to set up	Not achieved	Recall bias Sample not representative Incentives needed Group dominated by one participant

Working with a consulting firm specializing in customer surveys is one way to ensure the gathering of usable information (Sidebar 11.3). This will significantly increase the cost, but the facility benefits from the expertise of these specialists in both the questionnaire's design and analysis of the response data. Another alternative

SIDEBAR 11.3: Satisfaction Measurement Consultants

Measuring customer satisfaction in healthcare is big business and a number of experienced consulting firms are available from which to choose. Among the services they may offer are designing custom survey tools; organizing and facilitating focus groups; and conducting mail, telephone, and Internet-based surveys. With large databases of survey responses, these consultants may also provide market reports, goal-setting, and benchmarking support. Some limitations to consider when working with consultants are the method of data procurement, bias in interpretation, sample size, and resulting reliability.

Among the firms with national scope and a wide range of services are:

- Arbor Associates, Inc. (www.arbor-associates.com)
- Gallup (www.gallup.com)
- HealthStream Research (www.healthstreamresearch.com)
- Press Ganey Associates (www.pressganey.com)
- Professional Research Consultants, Inc. (www.prconline.com)

Table 11.2 Features of Quantitative Measurement Tools

Tool	*Cost Factors*	*Time line*	*Confidentiality*	*Risks*
Comment card	Low to moderate	May be ongoing; if one time, may be 1–2 months	Achieved, unless respondents identify themselves	Poor response Sample not representative Reflects high–low satisfaction
Mailed survey	Cost for representative sample high	1–2 months	Achieved, unless respondents identify themselves	Poor response Recall bias
Electronic survey	Less expensive than other survey types	May be ongoing; if one time, may be 1–2 weeks	Achieved if outside vendor used	Poor response Sample not representative
Telephone survey	Tends to be costly	Depends on sample size; 1–2 weeks minimum	Not achieved	Poor response Biased response Sample not representative
In-person interview	Relatively expensive for numbers reached	Immediate, if at time of service; 1–4 weeks otherwise	Not achieved	Biased response

is to use an existing survey that has been tested for reliability and validity (eg, Gallup poll) and make adjustments to meet the imaging facility's needs.

Survey methodologies vary and include a simple comment card given to patients following service, a questionnaire delivered via postal service or e-mail, and one-on-one interviews in person or by telephone. Selecting the appropriate tool is a key component in the process (Table 11.2). Regardless of the type, the survey can be a valuable conduit between stakeholders and the organization.

Comment Cards

Comment cards are among the least expensive ways to gather feedback from a specific group. Sized like a standard postcard, they usually consist of a few key questions or may simply ask the customer to provide feedback. They can be presented to customers at the time of service delivery with the options to complete the card immediately and drop it in an on-site response box or complete and mail it later.

The main advantages of comment cards are their low cost and ease of preparation. If questions are written correctly, the responses can be tallied over time and plotted on a bar graph to reveal frequency of negative and positive comments. When card comments are positive, these can be used in employee recognition activities.

On the other hand, the brevity of comment cards limits the variables that can be examined. Nor are the data statistically valid or random. Only 5% of patients will return a comment card, usually patients who are either very satisfied or very dissatisfied, making the sample unrepresentative of all patients.[1]

Mailed Questionnaires

Mailed questionnaires are a widely used methodology, primarily because there is no bias introduced by human interaction with the evaluation. A survey designed to be statistically reliable and valid and sent to a representative sampling of customers can collect satisfaction data that is quite valuable.

Mailed surveys must be visually appealing, easy to read, and so well designed that respondents can complete them without any questions or problems (see Box 11.1). Generally, questions fall within three categories: (1) factual (eg, patient age, date of visit, length of wait); (2) evaluative (eg, staff responsiveness, satisfaction with process); and (3) predictive (eg, likelihood of returning or of referring a friend).[1] Factual questions elicit information that can be useful in service planning and market segmentation; evaluations and predictions are the best measures of customer satisfaction (or dissatisfaction) and service quality.

Timing is a disadvantage of mailed surveys. Once the survey is created and the list of recipients compiled, several days are needed to ensure mail delivery. There is the lag time between service and survey completion, which may color the customer's responses due to lack of recall or intervening experiences. Questionnaires are also one of the most time-consuming measurement formats, a fact over which the sender has little control. The respondent may then take several days (or more) to complete the survey and the postal service more days to return it. Enclosing a postage-paid reply envelope and following up with reminder cards are ways to speed the survey return and increase the response rate.

Electronic Surveys

Sending a survey by e-mail or hosting one on the facility's Web site (see Box 11.2) is another way to speed the measurement process by eliminating the delivery time. Whereas once electronic surveys had not been a widely used tool for measuring satisfaction because of limited access to and comfort with the Internet by some categories of customers did not have or were reluctant to use it in this manner, thus affecting the representativeness of the sample. However, as computer usage has broadened and people have become increasingly accustomed to online communication, electronic questionnaires have become a popular alternative.

Box 11.1 Sample Patient Satisfaction Survey (mailed)

Patient Satisfaction Survey

We would like to know how you feel about the services we provide so we can make sure we are meeting your needs. Your responses are directly responsible for improving these services. All responses will be kept confidential and anonymous. Thank you for your time.

Your Age: _______

Your Sex:
Male ____
Female ____

Your Race/Ethnicity:
___ Asian
___ Pacific Islander
___ Black/African American
___ American Indian/Alaska Native
___ White (Not Hispanic or Latino)
___ Hispanic or Latino (All Races)
___ Unknown

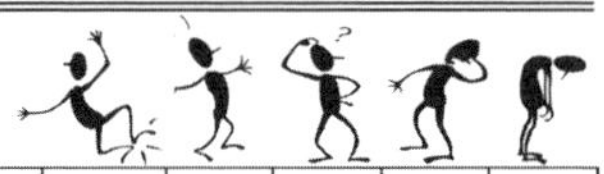

Please circle how well you think we are doing in the following areas:	GREAT 5	GOOD 4	OK 3	FAIR 2	POOR 1
Ease of getting care:					
Ability to get in to be seen	5	4	3	2	1
Hours center is open	5	4	3	2	1
Convenience of center's location	5	4	3	2	1
Prompt return on calls	5	4	3	2	1
Waiting:					
Time in waiting room	5	4	3	2	1
Time in exam room	5	4	3	2	1
Waiting for tests to be performed	5	4	3	2	1
Waiting for test results	5	4	3	2	1
Staff:					
Provider: (Physician, Physician Assistant)					
Listens to you	5	4	3	2	1
Takes enough time with you	5	4	3	2	1
Explains what you want to know	5	4	3	2	1
Gives you good advice and treatment	5	4	3	2	1
Radiation Technologists:					
Friendly and helpful to you	5	4	3	2	1
Answers your questions	5	4	3	2	1
All Others:					
Friendly and helpful to you	5	4	3	2	1
Answers your questions	5	4	3	2	1
Payment :					
What you pay	5	4	3	2	1
Explanation of charges	5	4	3	2	1
Collection of payment/money	5	4	3	2	1
Facility:					
Neat and clean building	5	4	3	2	1
Ease of finding where to go	5	4	3	2	1
Comfort and safety while waiting	5	4	3	2	1
Privacy	5	4	3	2	1

Confidentiality:					
Keeping my personal information private	5	4	3	2	1
The likelihood of referring your friends and relatives to us:	5	4	3	2	1
Do you consider this center your regular source of care?	Yes ____		No ____		

What do you like best about our center? ____________________

____

____

What do you like least about our center? ____________________

____

____

Suggestions for improvement? ____________________

____

____

Thank you for completing our Survey!

Source: U.S. Department of Health and Human Services, Health Resources and Services Administration. Available at: ftp://ftp.hrsa.gov/bphc/pdf/quality/patientsatisfactionsurvey.doc. Accessed March 25, 2009.

In addition to the much faster turnaround time, electronic questionnaires eliminate the expense of paper, printing, and postage. Another advantage over paper surveys is streamlined data analysis by software that links to the responses and automatically downloads them into charts and reports without the need for manual entry. The data are also more readily available in a user-friendly format to pinpoint trends and measure benchmarks. Response rates to electronic surveys can be unpredictable, and any e-mail addresses must be accurate and kept confidential.

In-Person Interviews

Formal, or in-depth, personal interviews can be conducted on site or off site, using a trained interviewer and a guide to provide structure to the interview. Ideally, the survey should be conducted after service has been provided to avoid bias resulting from a patient's reluctance to comment without anonymity while still undergoing care. Hiring a consultant interviewer who is not affiliated with the staff may increase a patient's willingness to give forthright comments. In some cases, patients may be willing to remain after a procedure to be interviewed, or with incentive, they may be willing to return to the office within a short period

Box 11.2 Sample Physician Satisfaction Survey (Web-based)

XYZ Imaging

Compassionate Care.
Reliable information.

About XYZ | Patient Guide | Physician Guide | News & Press | Contact

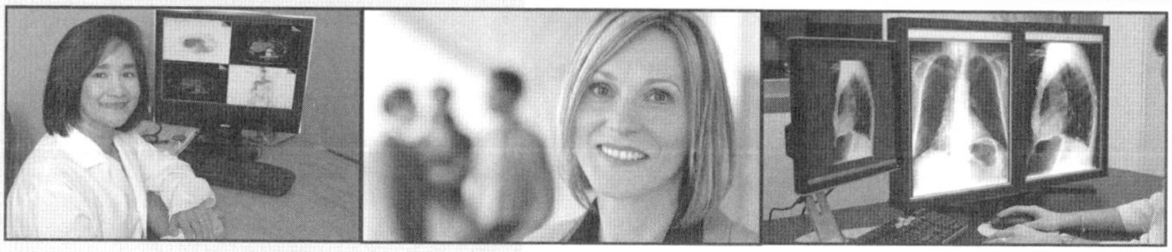

Physician Guide > Physician Satisfaction

Physician Satisfaction

Building and keeping your trust and confidence is extremely important to us. We strive to meet or exceed your needs and expectations in our patient care and communications. Please assist us to serve you better by completing the referring physician satisfaction survey and needs assessment. Thank you.

Please select the level of satisfaction that best reflects your experience:
1 = very dissatisfied, 2 = dissatisfied, 3 = neutral, 4 = satisfied, 5 = very satisfied, n/a = not applicable or unknown

Reports and Images	1	2	3	4	5	n/a
Accuracy of reports	○	○	○	○	○	○
Receive reports in a timely fashion	○	○	○	○	○	○
Radiologist calls when findings are significant	○	○	○	○	○	○
Ease of access to PACS	○	○	○	○	○	○
Quality of images	○	○	○	○	○	○
STAT readings (when requested) are prompt	○	○	○	○	○	○
Efficiency of film delivery	○	○	○	○	○	○

Quality of Professional Interpretations	1	2	3	4	5	n/a
CT	○	○	○	○	○	○
Mammography	○	○	○	○	○	○
MRI	○	○	○	○	○	○
Nuclear medicine	○	○	○	○	○	○
PET/CT	○	○	○	○	○	○
Ultrasound	○	○	○	○	○	○
Biopsy results	○	○	○	○	○	○

Customer Service	1	2	3	4	5	n/a
Phones answered promptly & minimal hold time	○	○	○	○	○	○
Level of knowledge/courtesy of office staff	○	○	○	○	○	○
Feedback from your patients about office staff	○	○	○	○	○	○
Feedback from your patients about the radiologist	○	○	○	○	○	○
Availability of urgent appointments	○	○	○	○	○	○
Days/hours of service adequate	○	○	○	○	○	○

Needs Assessment

	1	2	3	4	5	n/a
Accessibility of XYZ physicians	○	○	○	○	○	○
Personal interface with XYZ physicians	○	○	○	○	○	○
Availability of urgent and same day appointments	○	○	○	○	○	○
Quality of diagnostic equipment	○	○	○	○	○	○
Reputation of XYZ and physicians	○	○	○	○	○	○
Travel distance for patient	○	○	○	○	○	○

Overall Assessment

What does XYZ do best?

What does XYZ need to improve?

Check any of the following services if you were not aware they were offered by XYZ.

- ☐ Cardiac CT angiography
- ☐ Cardiac scoring
- ☐ MRA/CTA
- ☐ PET/CT
- ☐ CT virtual colonoscopy
- ☐ Nuclear medicine
- ☐ 3D/4D ultrasound
- ☐ Online reports

Submit

after the provided service. Waiting too long will introduce recall bias into their responses.

Compared with written surveys, a personal interview has the potential to acquire details that would not be forthcoming without the ability for the interviewer to ask probing follow-up questions. In this way, personal interviews have the potential to contribute both quantitative and qualitative data.

A form of personal interview can be effective in gauging referring physician satisfaction. After identifying the practices with the highest referral rates, as well as those that would be expected to refer but do not, the interviewer makes prearranged visits to each office to meet with one or more of the physicians and with staff members who interact with the imaging facility's staff. Using an interview guide, information can be gathered about what is the current level of satisfaction among referring practices, how the facility could change its procedures to solve identified problems or improve services, and why the non-referring practices recommend other facilities to their patients.

Following the interviews with patients or physicians, thank-you notes should be sent and any changes to be made as a result of their comments should be communicated.

Conducting personal one-on-one interviews can be relatively expensive, including the development of the guide, training the interviewer (or hiring a consultant), and the time needed for the interview and data analysis.

Personal Interview by Telephone

Telephone surveys are a popular means for measuring customer satisfaction, both of patients and referring physicians. Sharing many of the same advantages and disadvantages of in-person interviews, one of this tool's unique benefits is the ability to conduct the survey very shortly after the customer has been served. This decreases the likelihood of recall bias.

Among its unique drawbacks are: the number of contacts necessary to complete an interview, the short time frame to implement the phone contact, and the length of interview time.[1] These factors can influence the representativeness of the sample and bias the data. Research has found that making one attempt will reach just 24% of respondents; it may take up to 17 attempts to reach all respondents in the sample.[10] Calls are not scheduled, so there is no guarantee the responder is in the right position to accept the call and will be able to respond without emotion. If interrupted during dinner or another important time, the customer may project negative feelings onto his or her responses. If calls are made only on weekdays, the sample will be skewed toward retirees and the unemployed. Interviews lasting more than 15 minutes may cause fatigue or hostility that can bias subsequent responses.[11]

There are several factors to consider with this type of survey. Telephone interviews can be relatively costly to produce valid data. The questionnaire must be carefully designed, the interviewer(s) must be well trained to increase inter-rater reliability, the process of making calls and conducting interviews is time-consuming, and data must be analyzed. Hiring outside consultants to design, conduct, and analyze the survey is not likely to lower the cost but will help ensure statistically valid and reliable data from the effort.

Conclusion

The process of measuring customer satisfaction is complex but essential for imaging facilities. The many pieces of the survey process can only come together with sufficient resources, including adequate funding, visible support from senior management, and a willingness to participate from internal staff. The ongoing data accumulated from applying the various tools, as appropriate, are unavailable from any other source and will be invaluable in defining the organization's strategic objectives.

References

1. Ford RC, Bach SA, Fottler MD. Methods of measuring patient satisfaction in health care organizations. *Health Care Manage Rev*. 1997;22(2):74–89.

2. Van Campen C, Sixma H, Friele RD, Kerssens JJ, Peters L. Quality of care and patient satisfaction: a review of measuring instruments. *Med Care Res Rev*. 1995;52:109–133.

3. Leung FH, Savithiri R. Spotlight on focus groups. *Can Fam Physician*. 2009;55:218–219.

4. Barbour RS. The use of focus groups to define patient needs. *J Pediatr Gastroenterol Nutr*. 1999;28:S19–S22.

5. Tates K, Zwaanswijk M, Otten R, van Dulmen S, Hoogerbrugge PM, Kamps WA, Bensing JM. Online focus groups as a tool to collect data in hard-to-include populations: examples from paediatric oncology. *BMC Med Res Methodol*. 2009;9:15-22. Available at: http://www.biomedcentral.com/1471–2288/9/15. Accessed March 11, 2009.

6. Kenny AJ. Interaction in cyberspace: an online focus group. *J Adv Nurs.* 2005:49:414–422.

7. Im EO, Chee W. Issues in protection of human subjects in Internet research. *Nurs Res.* 2002;51:266–269.

8. Marx D. *Patient Safety and the "Just Culture": A Primer for Health Care Executives.* New York, NY: Columbia University; 2001. Available at: http://www.mers-tm.org/support/Marx_Primer.pdf. Accessed February 22, 2010.

9. Griffith KS. The growth of a just culture. *The Joint Commission Perspectives on Patient Safety.* 2009;9(12):8–9.

10. Naumann E, Giel K. *Customer Satisfaction Measurement and Management.* Milwaukee, WI: ASQ Quality Press; 1995:212.

11. Urden LD. Patient satisfaction measurement: current issues and implications. *Outcomes Manage.* 2002;6:125–131.

Chapter 12

Analyze and Apply Data

Kathy Tabor McEwan and Barbara Hubley

The true value of collecting customer satisfaction feedback lies in the ability to analyze and use the information to improve performance. Both qualitative and quantitative data lend themselves to analysis that can help the organization prioritize areas that will result in the greatest improvements in satisfaction. Efforts must also include activities that identify the key drivers of satisfaction and the root causes of dissatisfaction to ensure that scarce resources are applied in the most effective and efficient manner.

Because of the cost and effort involved, one estimate is that most businesses use less than half the customer information they collect and some use almost none of it.[1] Possible reasons for this gap between collection and implementation are both internal and external. First, the raw data may never be properly analyzed, since it is easier to collect customer information than it is to interpret it. Second, customer satisfaction consultants may analyze the data and produce a report, but they may believe that implementation is the client's responsibility. Third, the report may languish on the desk of the person who initiated the study with the results never passed on to the staff members best able to use them. Sometimes this is simply because the organization lacks effective communications and data sharing infrastructure; other instances may reflect poor management or judgment. However, simply measuring customer satisfaction will not contribute in a meaningful way to improving overall satisfaction.

Analyzing Satisfaction Data

If a facility has hired research consultants to conduct their customer satisfaction measurement program, it will receive one or more reports on a pre-determined schedule, in which the data will have been analyzed and graphically displayed. Depending on the contract, the consultant may also provide interpretation of the data and recommendations for implementation. It is important to have a basic understanding of how the data are processed; the availability of statistical software puts basic data analysis within the reach of non-specialists.

The progression from raw data to usable findings typically has four key steps:

1. Data are entered into a spreadsheet (Table 12.1). For electronic surveys and computer-aided telephone interviews, data entry is automatic. Measurement based on paper surveys or qualitative data will have to be entered manually.
2. Data are exported from the spreadsheet into a specialized statistical software program, which allows data to be analyzed using specified menu options.
3. The data input is checked carefully for errors, especially if data have been entered manually. These data undergo testing with various analytic processes (eg, cross-tabulating one response category to another or comparing averages) to produce the most useful results.
4. The results are formatted as graphs, tables, and charts, and depending on the intended audience, an accompanying narrative is written. Research consultants hired to conduct customer satisfaction measurement programs will produce one or more reports on a predetermined schedule, in which the data will have been analyzed, graphically displayed, and depending on the contract, interpreted as recommendations.

The second step is crucial: Understanding the tools available for "crunching the numbers" can allow a facility to broaden and deepen its investigation into customer satisfaction, permitting pinpoint findings. The techniques are designed to deal with the particular characteristics of qualitative and quantitative data, and to offer a range of pertinent conclusions.

Techniques to Analyze Qualitative Data

Qualitative research offers real benefits: An estimated 80% of improvement projects in businesses that have received the Malcolm Baldrige National Quality Award are the result of customer comments and suggestions.[2] Yet the thousands of customer words that can be generated by one or more qualitative tools can be overwhelming, even when the sample size is relatively small. Two analytic techniques can help organize and synthesize these data: cluster analysis and decibel analysis.

Cluster analysis (also called content analysis) aggregates the verbatim comments recorded during measurement into categories determined to be of interest (eg, convenience of service hours, staff professionalism). Researchers review all the comments and sort them into the categories and, if appropriate, subcategories. The interjudge reliability—the consistency determined by comparison of sorting decisions—is confirmed if at least 80% of the items match.

Table 12.1 Patient Satisfaction Survey Sample Data Collection Sheet

Question	*Great*	*Good*	*OK*	*Fair*	*Poor*	*No Response*
EASE OF GETTING CARE						
Ability to get in to be seen	40	44	16	0	0	0
Hours center is open	56	36	4	4	0	0
Convenience of center's location	48	44	4	0	4	0
Prompt return on calls	60	36	4	0	0	0
WAITING						
Time in waiting room	56	36	8	0	0	0
Time in exam room	56	44	0	0	0	0
Waiting for tests to be performed	40	56	4	0	0	0
Waiting for test results	40	56	4	0	0	0
STAFF - PROVIDER						
Listens to you	84	16	0	0	0	0
Takes enough time with you	80	20	0	0	0	0
Explains what you want to know	76	24	0	0	0	0
Gives you good advice and treatment	80	20	0	0	0	0
STAFF – TECHNOLOGISTS						
Friendly and helpful to you	84	16	0	0	0	0
Answers your questions	84	16	0	0	0	0
STAFF - ALL OTHERS						
Friendly and helpful to you	72	28	0	0	0	0
Answers your questions	72	28	0	0	0	0
PAYMENT						
What you pay is reasonable	48	44	8	0	0	0
Explanation of charges	48	44	8	0	0	0
Collection of payment/ money	48	44	4	0	0	4
FACILITY						
Neat and clean building	64	28	4	0	4	0
Ease of finding where to go	72	28	0	0	0	0
Comfort and safety while waiting	72	28	0	0	0	0
Privacy	60	36	0	0	0	4
CONFIDENTIALITY						
Keeping my personal information private	72	28	0	0	0	0
THE LIKELIHOOD OF REFERRING YOUR FRIENDS AND RELATIVES TO US.	72	20	0	0	0	8
DO YOU CONSIDER THIS CENTER YOUR REGULAR SOURCE OF RADIOLOGY CARE?	Yes - 91		No - 2		No Response - 7	

Source: U.S. Department of Health and Human Services, Health Resources and Services Administration. Available at: ftp://ftp.hrsa.gov/bphc/pdf/quality/patientsatisfactionsurvey.doc. Accessed March 25, 2009.

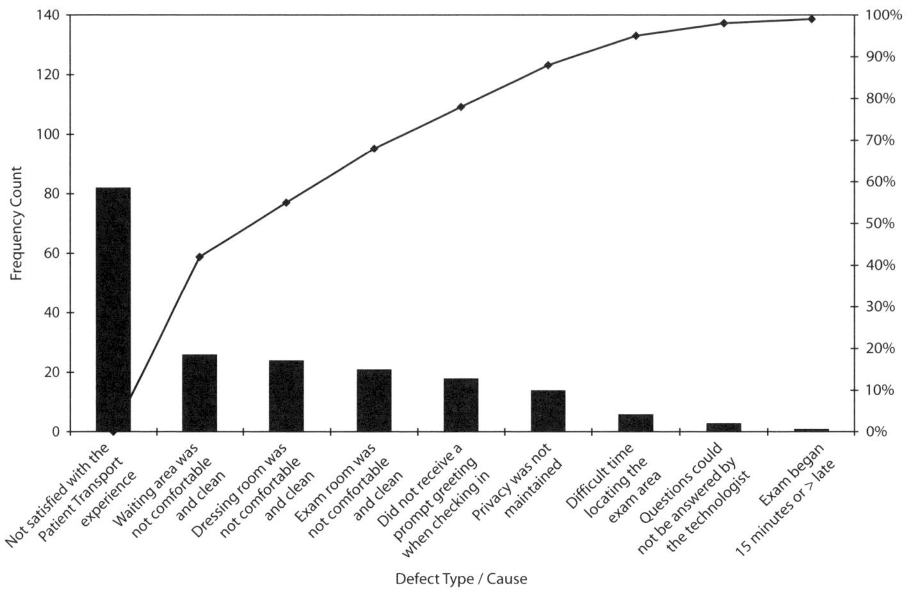

Figure 12.1 Pareto Chart

The results for each category can be graphically displayed as a Pareto chart (Figure 12.1). The horizontal x-axis presents the categories or key questions in descending order of frequency of customer responses. The left vertical y-axis usually represents number of responses and the right y-axis percentage of the total number of responses. A line graph superimposed over the bars represents the cumulative totals in each category. Pareto charts enable the user to quickly narrow the categories among the many comments to the few key features that should be addressed.

Further analysis of either positive or negative comments can be performed using decibel analysis with check sheets. Decibel analysis is designed to reflect the relative importance of a given feature to individual customers, which is lost when comments are aggregated into categories. The original responses are tallied onto a check sheet under a given category, and the customer's level of dissatisfaction (or satisfaction, in the case of positive comments/suggestions) is coded. The results, which are compiled into a table, help reveal the severity of dissatisfaction as it relates to one or more categories.

Techniques to Analyze Quantitative Data

The numerical nature of quantitative data lends itself to a variety of analytic techniques. Three of the most commonly used are (1) cross-tabulating; (2) frequency distribution; and (3) calculating and comparing means (averages).

Cross-Tabulating

Cross-tabulations allow comparisons of responses or demographics against other criteria or questions. For example, the administrator of an imaging center with

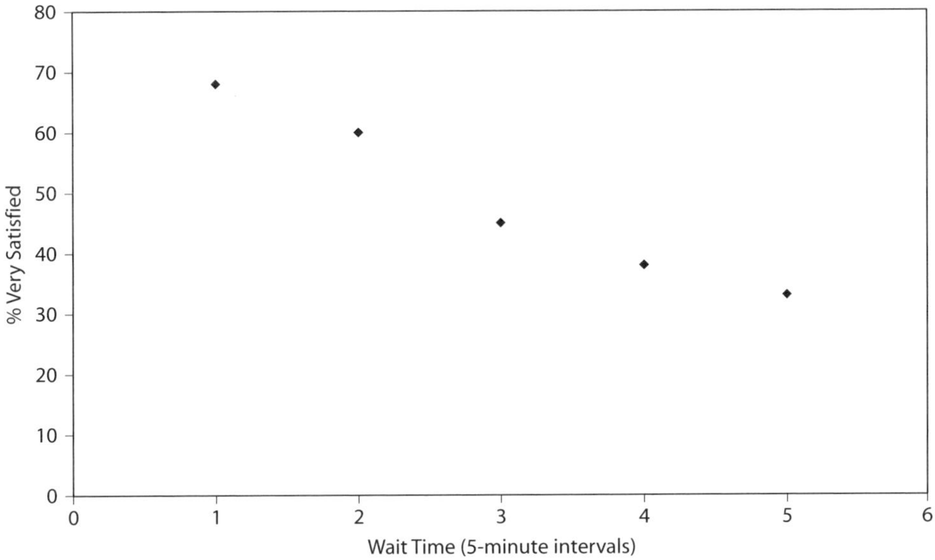

Figure 12.2 Relationship Between Wait Time and Satisfaction

multiple sites might want to compare responses on key satisfaction questions across all sites. The cross-tabulation would list the sites across the top, the key questions on the left, and the rankings by number or percentage of the ratings in the referent findings. As other examples, patients who rate the facility high in one category and also rate it high in another can be tracked; or one category of patients (eg, females) who consistently rate the facility higher on specified questions can be compared with another category of patients. In addition to being presented in a table, cross-tabulated data can also be displayed as a scatter graph (Figure 12.2).

The value of cross-tabulations lies in their simplicity and potential to reveal patterns of relationships in the variables. They do not explain, however, why the relationships exist.

Frequency Distribution

Results from surveys that use a scale (eg, very satisfied, somewhat satisfied) for responses can be analyzed using frequency distribution, rather than means and standard deviations. The response frequencies, usually expressed as percentages, are organized by category for each question (Table 12.2). Frequencies for key questions can be presented as pie charts (Figure 12.3). Over time, changes in these percentages can be tracked and presented as bar charts or line graphs, from which potential opportunities for improvement may be identified.

Table 12.2 Patient Satisfaction Survey Sample Frequency Table

Question	*Great*	*Good*	*OK*	*Fair*	*Poor*	*No Response*
EASE OF GETTING CARE						
Ability to get in to be seen	40%	44%	16%	0%	0%	0%
Hours center is open	56%	36%	4%	4%	0%	0%
Convenience of center's location	48%	44%	4%	0%	4%	0%
Prompt return on calls	60%	36%	4%	0%	0%	0%
WAITING						
Time in waiting room	56%	36%	8%	0%	0%	0%
Time in exam room	56%	44%	0%	0%	0%	0%
Waiting for tests to be performed	40%	56%	4%	0%	0%	0%
Waiting for test results	40%	56%	4%	0%	0%	0%
STAFF - PROVIDER						
Listens to you	84%	16%	0%	0%	0%	0%
Takes enough time with you	80%	20%	0%	0%	0%	0%
Explains what you want to know	76%	24%	0%	0%	0%	0%
Gives you good advice and treatment	80%	20%	0%	0%	0%	0%
STAFF - TECHNOLOGISTS						
Friendly and helpful to you	84%	16%	0%	0%	0%	0%
Answers your questions	84%	16%	0%	0%	0%	0%
STAFF - ALL OTHERS						
Friendly and helpful to you	72%	28%	0%	0%	0%	0%
Answers your questions	72%	28%	0%	0%	0%	0%
PAYMENT						
What you pay is reasonable	48%	44%	8%	0%	0%	0%
Explanation of charges	48%	44%	8%	0%	0%	0%
Collection of payment/money	48%	44%	4%	0%	0%	4%
FACILITY						
Neat and clean building	64%	28%	4%	0%	4%	0%
Ease of finding where to go	72%	28%	0%	0%	0%	0%
Comfort and safety while waiting	72%	28%	0%	0%	0%	0%
Privacy	60%	36%	0%	0%	0%	4%
CONFIDENTIALITY						
Keeping my personal information private	72%	28%	0%	0%	0%	0%
The likelihood of referring your friends and relatives to us.	72%	20%	0%	0%	0%	8%
Do you consider this center your regular source of radiology care?	Yes – 91%		No – 2%		No Response – 7%	

Source: U.S. Department of Health and Human Services, Health Resources and Services Administration. Available at: ftp://ftp.hrsa.gov/bphc/pdf/quality/patientsatisfactionsurvey.doc. Accessed March 25, 2009.

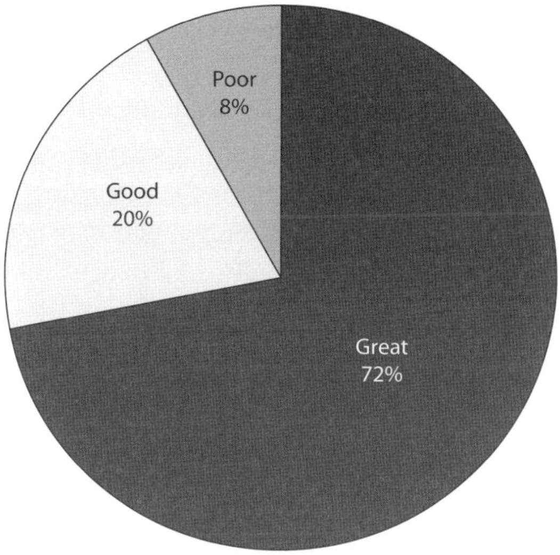

Figure 12.3 Likelihood of Patients to Refer Friends to Center

Comparing Means

The means, or arithmetic average, is calculated by adding all the values for a given set of responses and dividing by the number of responses. Standard deviation shows how much variation there is from the mean—a low standard deviation indicates that the data points tend to be very close to the mean, whereas high standard deviation indicates that the data are spread out over a large range of values. Comparisons are commonly made of means across time periods, groups of customers, or specific survey items. For example, the average wait time for the most recent quarter can be compared with that of the previous 8 quarters or the same quarter for the past 3 years. If a questionnaire asked patients to rate five attributes of the facility (eg, its parking convenience) on a 5-point Likert scale, the means of all responses for each attribute could be listed from highest to lowest. The relative importance of each attribute to the customer could be ranked by performing a paired t-test (using statistical software), which assesses whether the means of two groups are *statistically* different from each other. Means data can be presented in bar charts, line graphs, or tables, primarily based on personal preference.

Whatever analytic method is applied to the customer data, care must be taken to avoid jumping to conclusions about relationships, especially cause and effect. Statistical software can apply a number of tests to provide a measure of confidence in the probability that a given difference in the data reflects a true difference in the patient population. One or more of these tests should be performed before data are reported and actions are planned if costly mistakes are to be avoided.

Reporting Satisfaction Data

Imaging facilities have several categories of customers, including referring physicians, support services personnel, patients and their families, and even the facility's staff themselves. The various oversight staff in these areas each have an interest in receiving the results of customer satisfaction measures in a timely and effective fashion. Reports to senior management will usually focus on data relating to the entire organization, its overall business performance, and its competitive profile. The key attributes that scored well and those revealing opportunities for improvement should be highlighted.

Unit and area managers, and in turn, frontline employees should receive analyses of each item in the measurement tool, enabling them to participate meaningfully in devising goals and improving processes. Standard reports usually include customer participation rates, the overall facility rating, unit-specific results (eg, ultrasound, CT), and demographic data. Providing detailed data, rather than just aggregated measures, helps employees understand how each job contributes to overall customer satisfaction. If measurements are conducted on a regular basis, comparisons with previous data should also be provided to highlight trends.

"The transfer in pride in results comes when results are made visible."[2] Devising a visibility plan that includes not only communication but also recognition is important. Among its aspects should be:

- A procedure for how results will be reported, when, and by whom. This may include downloading results onto the facility's server for employees to access at their workstations, providing updates at regular staff meetings, or convening special meetings to review current results
- Data culled for opportunities to recognize as many employees as possible
- Publicizing of selected data: posted in public areas (those accessed by customers and employees), published in the facility's newsletter, and conveyed in letters to participating customers to broadcast results to the widest possible audience
- A process for keeping visible data fresh to avoid the impression of stagnation

Several formats for presenting data have already been described. In addition, tips for using specific visual formats include the following[3]:

- **Pie charts**: useful to depict any data that can be expressed as percentages, such as general performance or demographic information, and customer responses to global satisfaction questions

SIDEBAR 12.1: Organization of a Typical Report

Although ongoing surveys may only need relatively short reports, typically a report will be organized in the following fashion:

- Title page—includes the study topic, preparer, and date
- Table of contents—includes section titles and a list of charts and figures; the longer the report, the more detailed the table of contents should be
- Introduction and objectives—includes the basic purpose of the study, along with the specific objectives it was designed to meet; a brief description of methodology; and a summary of any limitations
- Executive summary—includes a concise, clear summary of the purpose, methodology, and findings, with enough detail provided to allow readers to accurately understand and use the study, even if they do not read the rest of the report
- Conclusions and recommendations—includes the preparer's conclusions and recommendations based on the results, outlined for potential managerial action
- Complete study findings—includes the details that support the preceding narrative sections, with relevant charts and graphs, organized in a logical fashion for ease of use
- Supporting charts and tables—includes the computer printouts of the data analyzed and the statistical processes used
- Appendices—includes additional material such as a copy of the questionnaire or more detailed statistical analysis

Source: Adapted from Stevens RE, Wrenn B, Sherwood PK, Ruddick ME. *The Marketing Research Guide*. 2nd ed. New York, NY: The Haworth Press; 2006:251

- **Mirrored bar charts**: useful to evaluate the relative importance of an attribute to customer satisfaction; these charts illustrate the fact that the lowest satisfaction survey scores are not necessarily associated with attributes that warrant the investment of resources toward improvement
- **Scatter graphs and quadrant charts**: used to facilitate prioritization of attributes for improvement efforts

Reports may be produced for a specific project (eg, in preparation for service changes), following an annual customer survey, or on an ongoing basis in conjunction with continuous customer satisfaction measurements. See Sidebar 12.1.

Using Satisfaction Data to Devise Organizational Goals

A five-step model that can guide an imaging facility's ongoing customer satisfaction program is as follows[4]:

1. Identify opportunities
2. Set priorities

3. Conduct root cause analysis
4. Design and test solutions
5. Implement solutions

Step 1: Identify Opportunities

It will be a rare organization that does not find multiple issues through customer satisfaction measurement. Faced with myriad data and reports, employees charged with improving satisfaction levels may feel compelled to address all the many issues at one time, perhaps with little success and a misuse of resources.

Therefore, it is worthwhile to establish criteria by which true opportunities can be identified. These criteria relate to scores that reflect a performance level below a baseline standard or show a significant deterioration over time. Each facility must set its own criteria, based on relevant benchmarks. For example, if a facility's survey asked respondents to use a 5-point scale of quality—excellent, very good, good, fair, or poor—an opportunity for improvement might be suggested by the following results: (a) an attribute rated "fair" or "poor" by more than 10% of respondents; (b) an attribute rated "excellent" by fewer than 40% of respondents; (c) a mean score below 4; or (d) a significant deterioration over time (as revealed by statistical analysis) in any one attribute's score.[4]

Step 2: Set Priorities

The number of legitimate opportunities identified in Step 1 will probably still be more than can be addressed at one time. It is important to prioritize these using qualitative and quantitative assessments. Consider both the importance to the customer as well as the likelihood of success while creating the prioritization. Two useful techniques are key driver analysis and constraint analysis.

Key Driver Analysis

This technique is a way to evaluate the importance of an attribute or opportunity to the customer in relation to the facility's performance. Customer survey responses that indicated the importance of specific attributes are subjected to regression analysis (Sidebar 12.2) to establish those that are most closely related to customer satisfaction.[3] These importance ratings are then ranked, as are the satisfaction ratings from the survey. A quadrant chart represents the findings (Figure 12.4), with the satisfaction values plotted on the x-axis from left being lowest to right the highest, and importance values on the y-axis with lowest on the bottom and highest at the top. Items appearing in the upper left quadrant (highest importance and lowest satisfaction) should receive priority attention because these issues are most important to customers but performance is currently unsatisfying to them. Correcting them will result in the greatest improvement in customer satisfaction levels.[5]

SIDEBAR 12.2: Regression Analysis

Regression analysis is a statistical tool used to establish the relationship of a dependent variable and one or more independent variables. By measuring exactly how large and significant each independent variable has historically been in its relation to the dependent variable, the future value of the dependent variable can be predicted. For example, an imaging facility may want to analyze its timeliness of appointments on customer satisfaction.

Using a technique called a scatter graph, it might plot on the X and Y axes the historical customer satisfaction scores for 10 years and the historical timeliness of appointments for the same period. A line connecting the average dots, called the regression line, would reveal the degree of correlation between the two factors by showing the amount of unexplained variation—represented by the dots falling outside the line. If the regression line connected all the dots, it would demonstrate a direct relationship between customer satisfaction and timeliness of appointments, meaning that one could be predicted on the basis of the other. The proportion of dots scattered outside the regression line would indicate, on the other hand, the degree to which the relationship was less direct, a high enough degree of unexplained variation meaning there was no meaningful relationship and that timeliness of appointments has no predictive value in terms of customer satisfaction.

Constraint Analysis

Another way to judge the importance of a given opportunity involves comparing the measure against various constraints, or markers of attainable performance. These include competitive constraints, benchmarks with similar facilities, historical values (eg, past results on the same measure), forecasts and trend analysis (especially for measures beyond the facility's control), and negotiated constraints

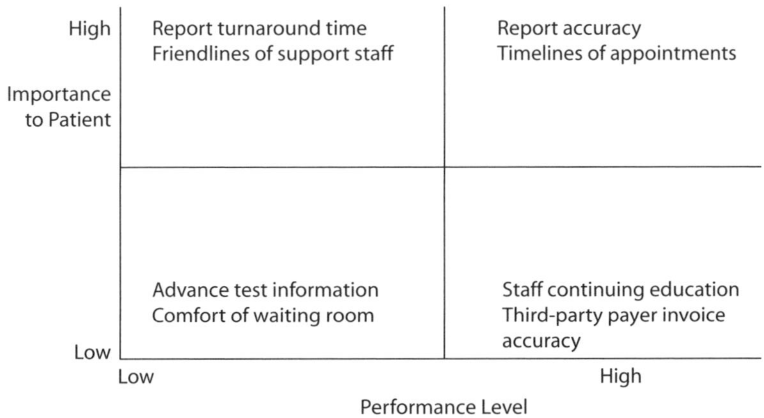

Figure 12.4 Quadrant Graph Depicting Relationship of Facility Performance on Attributes to Their Importance to Patients

(eg, with third-party payers).[6] The greater the gap between performance and the constraint, the greater the priority for change.

Step 3: Conduct Root Cause Analysis

Knowing what is important to customers and how the facility has performed are important to improving quality and satisfaction, but they are not enough. Too often at this point, the facility's staff will begin developing plans to correct deficiencies. Such actions are usually premature. Although staff members and managers may believe they know what has gone wrong and how to improve the situation, they are often unaware of the true, root cause of the customer's dissatisfaction and/or the deficient process. For example, if customers believe wait times are too long, what part of the process is the problem—with scheduling, the information they are given prior to arrival, the procedures of preparing patients for tests, or something else entirely? Root cause analysis can help clarify the key issues before valuable resources are spent.

The first step is to identify the opportunity that will be evaluated from the prioritized list. The next step is to carry out any additional research and analysis needed. In the example of excessive wait times, a flow chart of the patient appointment and check-in process can be created and the facility might record scheduling conversations for content review.

The third step involves creating an interview guide, listing several open-ended questions and concluding by soliciting patient suggestions for solutions to the problem. This guide is used to conduct a few random patient interviews or focus groups. For diagnostic purposes, only about 10 to 12 interviews usually need to be conducted.[4] These should be conversational (in person or by telephone) and timed to ensure the most accurate information about the issue being studied. Unlike the original satisfaction survey, these interviews are designed to elicit qualitative details; interviewers do not need to strictly follow the guide's questions but should probe each patient's responses for more details.

The fourth step involves organizing the information from the team's analysis and the patient interviews to identify themes. One way is to construct a list of common issues and suggestions, write each on a separate file card or small piece of paper, and sort similar ideas into piles, which will reveal themes or root causes.

Step 4: Design and Test Solutions

With the root causes revealed, potential solutions can be better assessed. Start by brainstorming a comprehensive list of alternatives, analyze the strengths and weaknesses of each, and discuss the preferred choices with key stakeholders before reaching a consensus on the first-choice option. If the solution involves significant changes in process or substantial investment of money or staff time, a pilot test is advisable. Testing on a small scale will provide insight into potential problems, help staff understand forthcoming changes, and ensure the final implementation will go smoothly.

Step 5: Implement Solutions

Section 4 details performance improvement methods that will help facilities implement solutions. Another book in this AHRA series, *Communication & Information Management in Radiology,* also discusses opportunity analysis as it relates to staffing, capacity, and other operational issues.

Conclusion

Ultimately, the activities of an imaging facility are focused primarily on patients, referring physicians, and their respective needs. Satisfaction data are invaluable resources that should be mined on an ongoing basis for insight into opportunities to address those needs in a manner that is superior to all other providers.

References

1. Denove C, Power JD IV. *Satisfaction: How Every Great Company Listens to the Voice of the Customer.* New York, NY: Portfolio; 2006:244.
2. Kessler H. *Measuring and Managing Customer Satisfaction: Going for the Gold.* Milwaukee, WI: ASQ Quality Press; 1996.
3. Naumann E, Giel K. *Customer Satisfaction Measurement and Management.* Milwaukee, WI: ASQ Quality Press; 1995.
4. Burroughs TE, Cira JC, Chartock P, Davies AR, Dunagan WC. Using root cause analysis to address patient satisfaction and other improvement opportunities. *Jt Comm J Qual Improv.* 2000;26:439–449.
5. Allen DR. *Customer Satisfaction Research Management.* Milwaukee, WI: ASQ Quality Press; 2004:160.
6. Griffith JR, White KR. *The Well-Managed Healthcare Organization.* 5th ed. Washington, DC: AUPHA Press; 2002:207.

4 Manage Performance Quality

In this section:

Chapter 13

Evaluate Continuous Quality Improvement Models

Jennifer Kroken

In its drive to achieve continuous quality improvement in performance, the healthcare industry has looked internally and externally for quality models. In particular, four of the most commonly used models that have been studied and adapted for application in both hospital and practice settings are: Total Quality Management, FOCUS-PDCA, Six Sigma, and Lean. Key elements of each, along with those of the Malcolm Baldrige National Quality Award, are discussed in this chapter.

Measuring customer satisfaction is an essential component of any imaging facility's drive to provide consistently high quality care. Accrediting agencies, third-party payers, and government oversight agencies have turned their focus to assessing quality, so no imaging facility can function without effective systems in place to measure performance and continuously improve patient care.

Among the challenges in measuring and improving quality in healthcare, however, are the questions of just what constitutes quality and who defines it. The US Agency for Healthcare Research and Quality has defined quality healthcare as "doing the right thing, at the right time, in the right way, for the right person—and having the best possible results."[1] The National Academies' Institute of Medicine definition is the "degree to which health services for individuals or populations increase the likelihood of desired health outcomes and are consistent with the current professional knowledge."[2] Both definitions, along with others, focus on outcomes as key indicators for quality. Other leaders in the field have suggested that quality incorporates the technical management of health and illness, the interpersonal relationship between providers and patients, the many amenities of care, and the underlying ethical principles that govern healthcare provision.[2]

Academics and agencies are not the only ones defining quality in healthcare. Customers have their own perceptions of quality of care. An imaging facility has several different categories of internal and external customers. While each shares a need and desire for quality, the definition of what constitutes that quality will vary from one group to another. Referring physicians will expect timely and meaningful reports detailing the patient's condition and a radiologist's call if an abnormality is found. The referring physician's office staff may evaluate quality in terms of the ease of working with an imaging facility's scheduling/registration staff. Patients will often judge quality based on the friendliness of staff during scheduling and registration; the comfort, cleanliness, and convenience (eg, ease of parking) of the facility; and supportive interactions with the technologist. Health plans judge quality based on access (that is, the availability of convenient appointment times), as well as accreditation or certification status.

From patient scheduling through performance of a procedure, imaging workflow can be broken down into a series of definable processes that impact overall quality. While today's quality improvement initiatives were developed in manufacturing environments, the principles of continuous quality improvement (CQI) have been shown to be applicable to almost every facet of imaging operations. (For more on the history of quality improvement, see another book in this AHRA series, *Communication & Information Management in Radiology*).

CQI approaches vary but virtually all are process oriented. Therefore, quality improvement tools can be used to improve a particular process in an operation whether it is reducing patient waiting times or increasing throughput. The key is isolating and identifying a problem in terms of its process steps. From there, the process needing improvement is defined and baseline performance levels are established. Performance levels are then tracked before, during, and after the initiative is implemented, so results can be identified and reported to accrediting agencies, patients, referring physicians, radiologists, hospitals, and the community at large.

In addition to their process orientation, the various quality improvement models share a number of other characteristics, including[2-4]:

- **An overarching belief that opportunity for improvement exists in every process on every occasion:** Continuous quality improvement is just that, continuous and ongoing, not a way to put out fires or a "flavor of the day" initiative.
- **A focus on overall or group performance rather than outliers:** It follows that these models are not about assigning blame and are instead nonpunitive, a quality that may be difficult to convince participants of in the early phases.
- **A focus on the customer:** Improvement projects are largely carried out based on their impact on the customer's perception of quality.

- **Data-based decision making:** What can be measured can be managed; information technology capabilities have significantly increased the ease with which data can be examined and presented to decision makers.
- **Employee empowerment:** Employees who are closest to the customer are often in the best positions to analyze processes and understand the impact on the customer; they will usually be the ones to implement process changes; and they must be authorized to make decisions that affect the customer experience.
- **Organization-wide commitment and leadership:** CQI programs are expensive in terms of both staff time and money, and cost savings are not always immediate or inevitable. In addition, these programs call for an organizational culture that embraces change (Sidebar 13.1). Senior management must be completely committed to the program and visibly demonstrate its commitment on an ongoing basis if employees are going to be willing to fully participate.

Healthcare has had quality assurance (QA) programs in place for a number of years and many facilities continue to carry out these activities. Like CQI, QA seeks to

SIDEBAR 13.1: Quality Leadership Is Change Leadership

Inherent in any continuous quality improvement effort is the need for changing the status quo. While some people are eager to initiate and embrace change, many others will resist. Managers who have led successful quality programs offer the following tips to develop a culture of change:

- Keep employees informed, starting well before the quality initiatives begin. Frequent communication should incorporate opportunities for open discussion and regular employee feedback.
- Put out a consistent, well-defined message, one that everyone agrees is worthwhile. It needs to be repeated often to all levels of the organization.
- Build continuing education programs into the plan. Supervisors may benefit from training in feedback and nonpunitive coaching skills. Staff will need specific training related to the changes.
- Fully inform and train supervisors and managers about the quality initiative, and enlist their support in its implementation, so they can in turn work confidently and reassuringly with staff.
- Give staff time to develop new skills and apply new procedures before the changes are incorporated into performance evaluations.
- Accept that some staff changes may be necessary for those who can not or will not adapt.

One resource for change management information and training is the Change Management Learning Center, www.change-management.com.

identify and eliminate process variation. It is the nature of that variation, however, that differentiates CQI from QA.

Processes have two primary types of variation: common cause (also referred to as systemic or internal variation) and special cause (or external variation). Common cause variation is usually random and is inherent in the process—it occurs as a result of the way in which the process is carried out. This variation can only be reduced by changing the underlying process itself. Special cause variation, on the other hand, is nonrandom variation that can be traced to a specific source. Eliminating this variation is usually possible once the source is identified.

QA focuses on eliminating defects or outcomes that result from special cause variation. Lacking a systemic or process-wide view, these activities may indeed eliminate a specific defect or variation, but they fail to take into account effects of the changes on other processes or parts of the system. Because CQI focuses on common cause variation, activities aim to eliminate or change entire defective processes and thereby control the variation. Recognizing the existence in healthcare systems of both forms of variation, CQI and QA programs are increasingly becoming combined; eliminating inappropriate variations helps managers predict performance. (For more about QA in imaging facilities, see the AHRA book *Asset Management in Radiology*.)

This chapter discusses the basic components of four quality improvement models that are commonly applied in healthcare and, specifically, imaging settings: Total Quality Management (TQM), FOCUS-PCDA, Six Sigma, and Lean.

Total Quality Management (TQM)

"TQM is a management philosophy that seeks to integrate all organizational functions ... to focus on meeting customer needs and organizational objectives."[5] It is more a person-focused premise than a systems overhaul approach. Developed in response to increasingly intense global competition in the mid-twentieth century, TQM sought to help U.S. companies shift from seeking the lowest cost methods to produce goods and services—which traditionally meant accepting a certain percentage of product "failures"—to focusing on producing quality goods and services and maximizing workforce effectiveness.[6]

The results of poorly performing processes are increased overhead, decreased revenue, and problems meeting service deadline requirements. TQM focuses on changing processes that are either outdated or hampering productivity, all with the goal of meeting customer expectations for quality and service. While improvements

Table 13.1 Traditional Organizational Attitudes Versus Those with TQM

Traditional	*TQM*
Other people are to be mistrusted.	Other people deserve our trust.
Blame others when things go wrong.	Work together to make improvements when things go wrong.
Life is competitive.	Life is cooperative.
Personal success is measured in competitive terms.	Success is measured in cooperative terms.
Problem solving is based on intuition and gut feelings.	Problems are analyzed and solutions are based primarily on data.
Individuals who are good at "putting out fires" are the champions.	Teams who can prevent fires are honored.
Rewards are finite; one employee's gain is another's loss.	Cooperation leads to rewards, growth, and potential gains for all.

Source: Adapted from Capezio P, Morehouse D. *Taking the Mystery Out of TQM: A Practical Guide to Total Quality Management*. Franklin Lakes, NJ: Career Press; 1995:180–181.

in quality occur incrementally by improving one process at a time, TQM is not simply a single "process fix" but a performance improvement philosophy that ultimately transforms how business is conducted.

The many facets of TQM may seem overwhelming. Physicians, senior management, and staff must be solidly committed to make it happen. No department is exempt from scrutiny for ways to improve. Many organizations have found that once they take on a TQM program and begin to see improvement, excitement builds and employees become very proud of the fact that they work for a quality company (Table 13.1). TQM is a top-to-bottom effort in that it involves all levels of employees.

Healthcare and other organizations that successfully implement TQM share the following characteristics[7]:

- They are customer driven with a focus on total customer service.
- They take a long-term view of their business, rather than focus on short-term profitability.
- They are continuously improving their staff, their processes, and their service.
- They seek out and eliminate waste.
- They create quality at the source, rather than inspecting for quality after the fact.
- They encourage high employee participation in all aspects of the organization, with multilevel communication, cross-functional teams, and managers who coach and mentor employees. (For in-depth discussion of these strategies, see the AHRA book *Human Resource Management in Radiology*.)

Three commonly implemented TQM programs are Socio-Technical Systems, Statistical Process Control, and Just-in-Time.

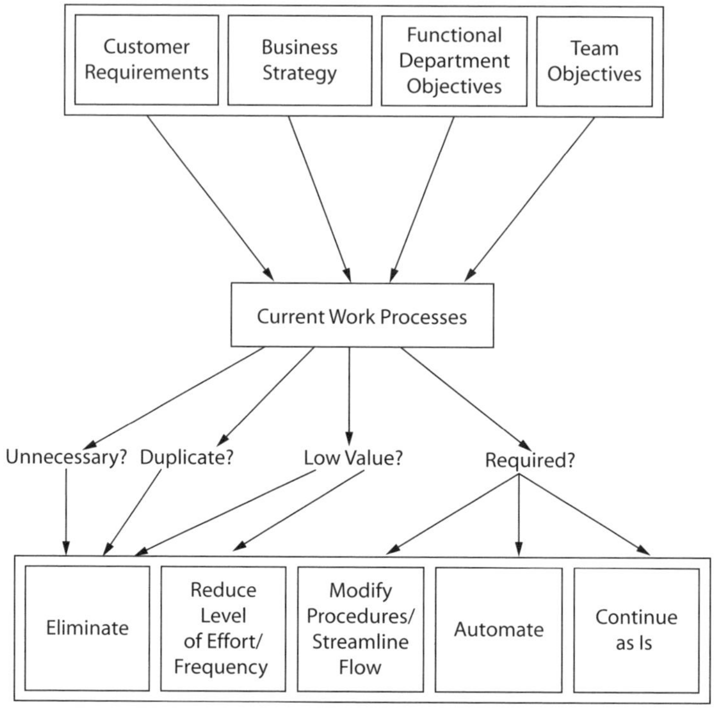

Figure 13.1 Analysis of Current Work Processes Based on Key Influences

Source: Adapted from Capezio P, Morehouse D. *Taking the Mystery Out of TQM: A Practical Guide to Total Quality Management*. 2nd ed. Franklin Lakes, NJ: Career Press; 1995:243.

Socio-Technical Systems

Employee empowerment, one of the guiding principles of TQM, arises out of research showing that when workers are allowed to participate in the design of workplace changes, productivity increases.[7] The Socio-Technical Systems program examines how well the social system (ie, the interface between people) and the technical system (ie, the workplace technology) are designed to work with each other and to meet customer needs. As program participants seek to identify work processes to improve, no process is viewed in isolation from the organization as a whole (Figure 13.1). Work functions are examined closely to eliminate redundancy, with the view that all work should add value to the work of others and to the final service/product.

In trying to identify work processes to improve, many organizations follow these steps[7]:

1. Key processes are identified.
2. Data are collected and analyzed, using either existing measures or ones created for the project.
3. The current situation is defined.

4. The ideal situation is defined.
5. The ideal situation is pilot-tested within a subgroup.
6. The results of the pilot test are analyzed, any necessary changes are made, and if needed, a second pilot test is carried out.
7. A cost-benefit analysis is carried out on the pilot test results.
8. The pilot test results and cost-benefit analysis are presented to decision makers for organization-wide implementation.

Statistical Process Control

Another guiding principle of TQM focuses on identifying and eliminating variance in processes as a means to achieve quality. One of the primary ways this is accomplished is with Statistical Process Control, a program that aims to achieve conformance to agreed-on specifications, remove unacceptable variation, and keep processes within established tolerances or standards (ie, best practices). Although developed for a manufacturing environment, Statistical Process Control can also be applied to services such as healthcare.

This is a data-intensive program. A good starting point is a problem area identified by a customer satisfaction survey, a process that lends itself to quantitative measurement, or one that is crucial to the success of a specific unit. Data, either historical or current, should be collected over a predetermined time period and plotted on a control chart, scatter diagram, or other graph. Review of the charts, often accompanied by a flow chart of the process, will help identify trends that can be analyzed for root cause(s) and ultimately changes to the process to bring the results within the standards.

The control charts in Figures 13.2, 13.3, and 13.4 show three circumstances that suggest processes may be out of control and need further analysis. A shift (Figure 13.2) occurs when at least seven consecutive data plot points fall above or below the average (center line). A trend (Figure 13.3) is revealed when six or more consecutive data plot

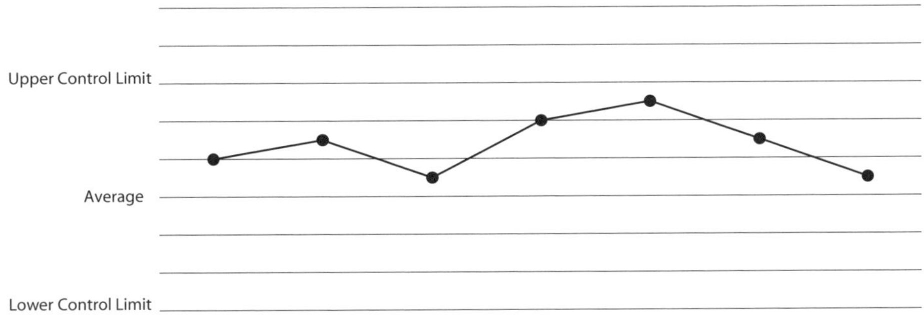

Figure 13.2 Control Chart Showing Data Shift Indicating Out-of-Control Process

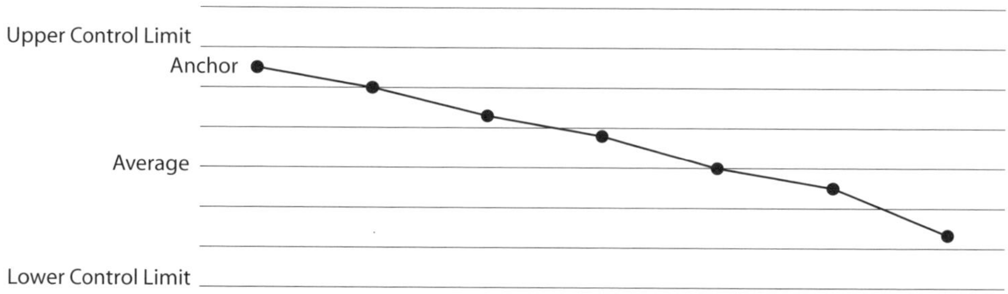

Figure 13.3 Control Chart Showing Data Trend for Potential Out-of-Control Process

points move up or down from a single anchor point. A jump (Figure 13.4) is the change between two consecutive plot points that is at least two-thirds the distance between the upper and lower limits.

Just-in-Time

Just-in-Time programs aim to eliminate waste, continuously improve procedures, produce goods or services based on demand, and ensure that each step in a process is carried out with 100% accuracy. As with other quality efforts, the program has numerous components to achieve these goals, among which are the use of improvement teams, the development of strategic vendor relations, and a focus on individual responsibility for quality.[7]

Improvement teams involve employees at all levels with the change process. These teams often focus on a specific area (eg, safety standards compliance or productivity improvements). Trained in problem solving, consensus building, and team dynamics, members use techniques including brainstorming, data analysis, and process analysis to encourage new ways of thinking about commonly performed tasks.

One of the most popular areas for Just-in-Time programs in healthcare has been in vendor relations and related inventory management. The program's approach is to build long-term relationships with single-source suppliers that commit to providing

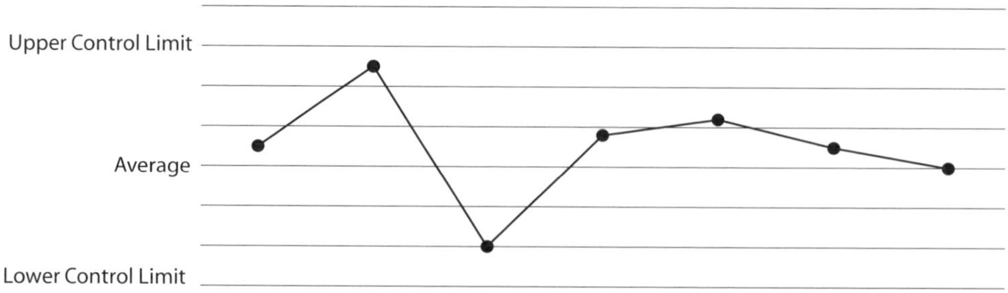

Figure 13.4 Control Chart Showing Data Jump for Potential Out-of-Control Process

the highest quality items while continuously seeking to reduce costs. Emphasizing quality throughout the supply chain reduces the need for the practice to inspect goods and the likelihood that defects will occur to affect patient care. In some instances, suppliers are asked to warehouse high-priced, low-demand items and ship on consignment as needed, lowering practice inventory costs and potential waste. Negotiating best prices with a single source allows organizations to streamline their ordering processes. A Seattle medical center, for example, instituted a system that puts a reminder card at the bottom of a set of supplies to signal the need to reorder, helping lower inventory costs by $1 million.[8] An academic practice of 11 physicians saved $88,000 on office supplies while serving 715 more patients in a single year by canceling standing delivery orders and lowering on-hand inventory to a 1-week's supply in examination rooms and a 4-week's supply in a new controlled-access central supply room.[9]

A fundamental concept of Just-in-Time is that each operation or department must view the next operation or department as its customer and therefore must strive to achieve error-free service. In TQM terminology, this is referred to as quality at the source. Employees are recognized as trustworthy and knowledgeable about the processes and services they provide. Managers serve as coaches and mentors who must relinquish some of their day-to-day control to the employees, who are encouraged to intervene if a process is defective (eg, an error occurs). Employee suggestion and recognition programs are traditional activities that are incorporated into the Just-in-Time toolkit.

The FOCUS-PDCA Cycle

As with many other quality improvement models, the Plan-Do-Check-Act (PDCA) cycle was created to make changes to manufacturing processes. In the 1980s Hospital Corporation of America modified the process to reflect the tasks that needed to be carried out before the PDCA cycle could be implemented. The modified version is called the FOCUS-PDCA cycle (Figure 13.5) and is now the most commonly applied quality improvement model in healthcare in the United States.[2] FOCUS is the acronym for its five steps: find, organize, clarify, understand, and select.

Begin to FOCUS

Find the Problem

The cycle begins with the identification of a process to improve. Customer complaints, staff suggestions, and brainstorming sessions are just a few of the ways to identify problems that might be tackled. The list can be narrowed by selecting a

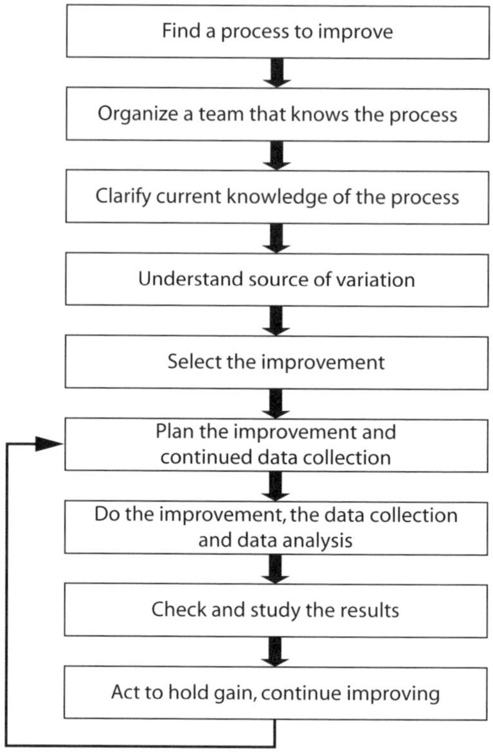

Figure 13.5 FOCUS-PDCA

problem that affects customer satisfaction, will show a return on investment if eliminated, or is perceived to be amenable to change. For example, a hospital might complain of slower imaging report turnaround following implementation of voice-activated dictation, which is contrary to expectations. The definition (or "find") of the problem is slow report turnaround.

Organize a Team

A team needs to be organized to fix the problem. An effective team will have representatives from three groups: stakeholder categories affected by the process under review; staff directly involved with and knowledgeable about the current process; and a resource person who is experienced in CQI to train the other team members and facilitate their activities. In the example of the slow report turnaround, the team would include a radiologist, a technologist, administrative personnel responsible for ensuring the referring doctors get their reports, and perhaps someone from information technology services.

Clarify Current Processes

The team must clarify what the current process is before any changes can be made. Flowcharting can be extremely useful at this stage, if not critical, and may take more than one meeting to complete. One technique is to have several team members each prepare a flowchart, then compare the documents. Any variations will be revealed and may identify areas for change. The flowchart also helps the team assess whether the scope of the process makes it suitable for improvement.

Understand Sources of Variation

The team must understand the causes of the process variation before devising a plan to eliminate it. This entails identifying relevant quality measures, collecting valid and reliable data about current process performance, and analyzing the data. In some cases, measures may already exist and data have been collected; the team only needs to access the data, document the level of variation based on those data, and identify the causes of the variation. In other cases, new measures may have to be devised and data collected before the team can begin to analyze the variation and its cause(s). For the slow report turnaround example, a review of daily report logs may reveal that two radiologists account for 90% of the delayed reports and those radiologists edit their reports at the end of their shift, rather than as the test results become available.

Select a Process to Improve

The team evaluates and selects the process improvement plan. Because most problems will have various possible solutions, the team should devise selection criteria, which characterize the improvement plan in terms of time needed to implement, the costs, the feasibility, and/or the likelihood of resistance by key players. Each potential improvement plan is assessed based on the criteria and one is selected, initiating the PDCA part of the cycle.

The PDCA Component

Plan

Now that the team has direction, it can devise a plan of action to fix the problem. This step involves translating the improvement plan into specific actions that identify who will carry out the improvement pilot, what specific changes are to be piloted, and how success will be measured.

Do

During this second step, the agreed-on plan is implemented in a pilot test phase, and any deviations (defects) in the expected outcome are documented. If needed, equipment is modified or installed, involved staff members are trained, and tools are put in place to measure results. New procedures are documented for future use. For the example of the slow report turnaround, having identified end-of-shift report preparation by two radiologists as the primary cause of the delays, the plan might involve meeting with the physicians, discussing their work habits, and cultivating their commitment to a trial of preparing reports as test results become available.

Check

This may be the most important stage in the PDCA cycle. More data gathering is in order, using Pareto charts, control charts, and other tools, to evaluate what went right, what went wrong, and whether another test cycle is needed. If so, the team also needs to decide on any changes in the improvement plan and whether additional training is necessary. In the example, if changing the radiologists' work habits does not improve the overall report turnaround time as expected, the team must review the plan, analyze why it failed to produce the desired results, and implement another test.

Act

Finally, the team determines the success of the plan and makes one of several decisions: adopt the plan, adjust it, or abandon the plan completely. If the team decides to adopt the plan, the new procedures and quality measures need to be documented and all staff trained. If the pilot test in the report-turnaround example met with success, then a meeting with the entire clinical staff may be in order so all radiologists are made aware of the desired workflow. Results must continue to be monitored so gains are not lost. There should also be a person assigned to continually track report turnaround time so the hospital is not the one to notify the department of future problems. Then a new problem can be undertaken and the FOCUS-PDCA cycle can begin again.

As with most CQI programs, FOCUS-PDCA is an evolving phenomenon whereby processes are continually changing and therefore must be monitored. Operations managers may find while working on their tenth process improvement initiative that the first process improvement initiative just slipped back into problem status. Continual monitoring of improvements is necessary for the success of the program.

The Six Sigma Model

Six Sigma, created by Motorola and successfully adopted by GE and other major corporations, is a statistics-based model that focuses on redesigning processes to eliminate defects. In healthcare, those defects include medical errors, delays, and costly mistakes. Six Sigma "provides specific methods to re-create the process so that defects and errors never arise in the first place," a departure from quality-control programs that focus on detecting and correcting defects as they arise.[10]

Table 13.2 Rate of Defects per Sigma

Sigma	*Defects/Million Opportunities*	*Example: No. Prescription Errors/Year*
2	308,537	6,170,740
3	66,807	1,336,140
4	6210	124,200
5	233	4660
6	3.4	68

Source: Adapted from Harry M, Schroeder R. *Six Sigma*. New York, NY: Currency/Doubleday; 2000.

A sigma in statistics represents standard deviation from the norm. When applied to defects per million opportunities, a higher sigma equals a lower rate of defects and thus a more efficient process. Table 13.2 shows that at six sigma, the rate of defects is reduced to about 3.4 defects per million, an accuracy rate of about 99.99%.[11]

The Six Sigma model can be applied to a wide range of projects within healthcare. For imaging facilities, Six Sigma has been used to[12]:

- Reduce the incidence of patient falls
- Improve the revenue cycle
- Increase employee retention
- Decrease the number of lost films
- Improve examination scheduling

Mikel Harry and Richard Schroeder, who led Motorola's Six Sigma initiative, argue that the highest quality results in the lowest costs,[10] which has been borne out by not only major corporations but also healthcare facilities. One Kentucky hospital reduced its annual imaging expenses by $800,000 and errors in the magnetic resonance ordering process by 90% within 18 months of implementing a Six Sigma program.[13] For patients who required diagnostic follow-up after a screening mammography, a Florida breast care center was able to reduce the time from a patient's initial call for an appointment for screening mammography to delivery of her biopsy results from 13 weeks to just 3 weeks. The change not only increased patient satisfaction, but also created 10% more appointment slots, eliminated rework on subsequent appointments, and enabled the purchase of an additional digital mammography unit.[14]

While Six Sigma can be applied to any sized business, the high volumes in imaging make the model a particularly good fit. For example, if a 12-person imaging group reads 240,000 examinations per year (20,000 per person) and each examination involves both a primary and a secondary insurer, then the billing transaction count is 480,000. If a billing office functions at the three sigma level, the practice could see more than 32,000 billing errors annually.

The Six Sigma Process

Six Sigma requires a full-time commitment by either a consultant or a trained in-house expert to identify projects, train staff in Six Sigma methodology, and facilitate project teams. Projects are carried out using six steps, designated by the acronym DMAIC: define, measure, analyze, improve, and control. In the discussion below, each step is applied to a hypothetical project to reduce insurance denials in an imaging billing office.

Define

The first phase in Six Sigma is to define the project by creating a project charter. This document outlines the customer need(s) that the project is designed to fulfill; the project scope, goals, success criteria, team members, available resources; any constraints (eg, no new hires); and rough deadlines. Before work begins on the project, this document should be presented to the facility's leadership team and authorization received. Six Sigma projects require major investments in time and money and should only be initiated with solid management support. If this is the first Six Sigma project, the charter can also be used in the request for proposal if a consultant is to be hired to facilitate the project or in the job description for an in-house expert.[15]

In the case of the hypothetical billing office discussed above, the project would seek to reduce the rate of insurance claim denials from 14% to less than 5% within 6 months of implementing the project. While no new staff can be hired, technology upgrades can be considered. The project team, which will be led by a Six Sigma consultant, will include the billing supervisor, a billing clerk, a financial analyst, an information technologist, and a front-office staff member.

Measure

Six Sigma is a data-driven model, making this step especially crucial. The appropriate metrics for the project must be identified; they must be reliable and valid; and a process must be in place to measure them before, during, and after the project. Criteria for progress and for success should be specified. Also at this step, data are collected that clarify the depth of errors or defects currently in the system.

A review of claims for the past 3 months in the hypothetical billing office found 900 denials in 6500 claims, which were categorized into nine categories (Figure 13.6). The same data were also categorized by insurance carrier (Figure 13.7). The relative frequency of each category was then calculated (Tables 13.3 and 13.4).

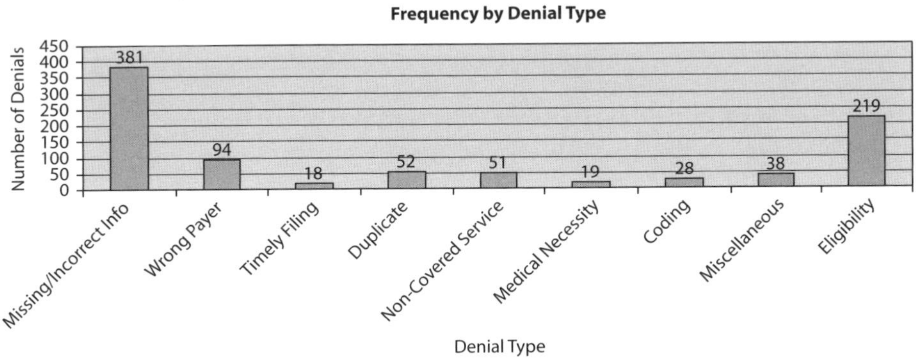

Figure 13.6 Frequency of Claims Denial by Type in Hypothetical Imaging Facility

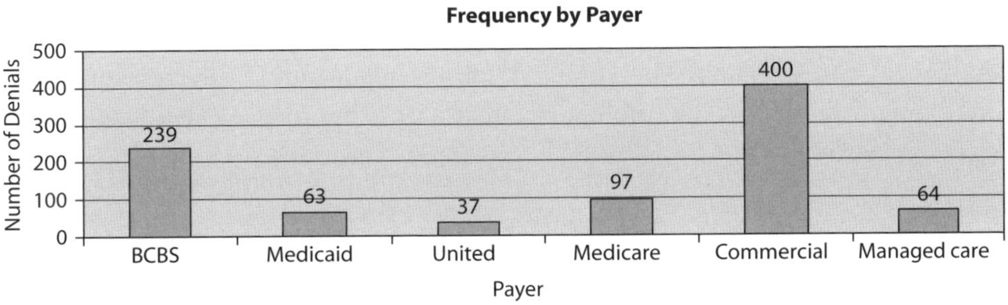

Figure 13.7 Frequency of Claims Denial by Insurance Carrier in Hypothetical Imaging Facility

BCBS indicates Blue Cross Blue Shield.

Table 13.3 Frequency of Claim Denial by Reason for Denial in Hypothetical Imaging Facility

	Frequency	*Relative Frequency (rounded to nearest hundredth)*
Missing/incorrect information	381	.42
Wrong payer	94	.10
Timely filing	18	.02
Duplicate	52	.06
Non-covered service	51	.06
Medical necessity	19	.02
Coding	28	.03
Miscellaneous	38	.04
Eligibility	219	.24
Total	900	1.00

Table 13.4 Frequency of Claim Denials by Insurer in Hypothetical Imaging Facility

Insurer	*Frequency*	*Relative Frequency (rounded to nearest hundredth)*
Blue Cross Blue Shield	239	.27
Medicaid	63	.07
United Healthcare	37	.04
Medicare	97	.11
Commercial	400	.44
Managed care	64	.07
Total	900	1.00

Relative frequency is calculated by dividing the number of occurrences in a particular category by the total number of occurrences (eg, denials for missing/incorrect information appeared 381 times in Table 13.3, divided by 900, the total number of the denials). The total relative frequency must always equal one. Compiling data graphically into control charts or other formats will facilitate the next step, analysis.

Analyze

In addition to carefully analyzing the data control charts, the project team may need to prepare a process map or flowchart to identify specific areas of process variation. This step also seeks to clarify the degree to which the process deviates from standards, whether the process is amenable to improvement, and what resources will be needed. Various hypotheses about the source(s) of the variation may need to be tested.

In the example under consideration, the commercial insurance category overwhelmingly accounts for the largest proportion of denials (Table 13.4). This category, however, includes hundreds of insurance companies, each of which accounts for five or fewer claims per month, making this category an almost impossible one to target for a Six Sigma project. Therefore, the team focuses on the next highest frequency, Blue Cross Blue Shield, recognizing that any specific actions taken to eliminate Blue Cross Blue Shield denials are likely to have a positive impact on other insurance classes as well.

Reviewing Table 13.3, the team also notes that missing/incorrect information as a reason for denial has by far the largest frequency. A flowchart identifies several areas that represent likely sources for missing or incorrect information, beginning with scheduling and registration. Patients may provide incorrect insurance information because they are unaware of a plan or policy change. Another possibility identified occurs when front desk personnel do not consistently verify patient information or are inadequately trained. The analysis may take several attempts to find the source(s) of the bad information.

Improve

At this stage, the team should be ready to design and implement the needed process changes to ensure performance improvement. Six Sigma encourages and empowers employees to repeatedly examine what they do and how they do it and ask, "Is there a better way?" Although solidly based on data and goals, the implementation plans may call for creativity and risk-taking, especially if significant sigma improvements are needed. A process that is operating at four sigma cannot be brought to six sigma simply by tweaking it.

In the example, the team discovers that the patient registration software has an option that provides on-screen reminders for key information and can be programmed to prevent screen closure if information is missing. The upgrade is purchased and installed; front-desk staff are trained and monitored. In addition, a lunch-and-learn session is held for billing and front-desk staff with a Blue Cross Blue Shield representative to highlight the company's procedures and answer questions.

Control

"The primary reason for undertaking a Six Sigma project is to change the status quo.... In a Six Sigma project, change is inevitable."[15] Change is rarely easy or straightforward, so the final step in the Six Sigma model is designed to ensure that changes for the better are retained over the long run, until new technology or other factors call for another assessment. Management must put new policies and procedures into place, and train and support employees during the transition period. Quality controls and possibly new metrics must be developed to allow ongoing monitoring of the new process.

The hypothetical team continued to review denial data for several months during which the overall denial rate dropped to the target 7%. A report of the denial rate was added to monthly staff meetings, so all staff members would be reminded of the benefits of the new procedures.

The Lean Model

While Six Sigma focuses on defects and quality, Lean concentrates on reducing time, costs, and waste, all of which are components of performance. Developed by Toyota Motor Corporation, its principles are informed by the philosophy that an ideal system should be simple, always acknowledge room for improvement, and continuously get better.

Lean broadly defines waste—also known as non-value-added activities—as anything that does not enhance the customer's experience, motivate the customer to buy, or contribute to the financial success of the business. There are seven types of waste[16] (listed here with examples from an imaging business):

1. Overproduction (unnecessary tests)
2. Inventory (excess supply inventory)
3. Defects (poor quality films)
4. Motion (poor workstation ergonomics)
5. Waiting (poor patient scheduling)
6. Overprocessing (outdated procedures)
7. Transport (poor patient flow)

Lean and Six Sigma differ in a number of key ways[17]:

- While Six Sigma projects are often complex and take months to complete, Lean focuses on simpler projects that may take as little as a week to carry out.
- Six Sigma relies on problem-solving statistical techniques to achieve its results; Lean teaches several basic principles and applies best practices.
- Six Sigma calls for dedicated resources and organization-wide training; Lean uses short workshops on an as-needed basis.

Despite their differences, or perhaps because of them, Six Sigma and Lean are increasingly used simultaneously, especially in healthcare. Because of the speed with which most Lean projects can be carried out, tackling a few at the start of a quality initiative can build momentum for the subsequent, more complex Six Sigma projects.

Lean methods incorporate the use of *kaizen*, a Japanese term which simply means "continuous improvement" and is a fundamental part of this quality model. In the recent past, Lean and kaizen have in some circles become separated initiatives, whereas they are really intertwined concepts. The term "Kaizen Event" (or a "Kaizen Blitz") further complicates this relationship; however, it is essentially an extension of the same model and is the rapid-change event(s) designed to test improvements. It is commonly understood to have a simple tactical focus, and key characteristics include: short duration (1–6 days), intense focus, a sequestered team, the involvement of all stakeholders, facilitation (not leading), aggressive goals, low cost, rapid decisions, and immediate implementation and training.

Value Stream Mapping

The most commonly used Lean tool, value stream mapping, can be useful in identifying projects, some of which are best carried out using Six Sigma techniques.

Value stream mapping is a visual tool that helps gain understanding of the flow of material and information as a product or service makes its way through the value stream. It differs from the process mapping of Six Sigma in four ways[18]:

1. It gathers and displays a far broader range of information than a typical process map.
2. It tends to be at a higher level (five to ten boxes) than many process maps.
3. It tends to be used at a broader level, that is, from receiving of raw material to delivery of finished goods.
4. It tends to be used to identify where to focus future projects, subprojects, and/or kaizen events.

A value stream map takes into account not only the activity of the product or service, but the management and information systems that support the basic process. This is especially helpful when working to reduce cycle time, because insight is gained into the decision-making flow in addition to the process flow.

The basic idea is to first map the process, then above it map the information flow that enables the process to occur. A set of specific symbols is used in creating the map, making it look confusing and haphazard to the untrained observer. The steps in the process occupy the center of the map; information flowing in and out of the process appears at the top. Along the sides and bottom are boxes with relevant data. The map also includes a timeline that incorporates both wait and process times. See Figure 13.8 for an example of a "current state" and "future state" value stream map.

Initially, the map is created with paper and pencil; once the quality team agrees on its accuracy, software is available to produce a more polished version for ongoing use. Some teams find it useful to have several team members each produce a map, then identify areas of disagreement for further discussion and possible data collection. The team highlights specific areas on the map that will be the focus of quality improvement projects.

Once a facility has established its vision and strategic goals for the quality initiative, the Lean model follows this sequence[19]:

1. Identify the value stream, the area that will be the focus of the quality effort; Pareto charts based on volume or other data are a useful tool to pinpoint the service line that is likely to benefit from the attention.
2. Identify and collect initial metrics related to the value stream, including existing past data and, if necessary, data collected specifically for the initiative.

Total Process Time	50 min
Value Added Time	18 min
Wait Time Range	3.5 hours –10 days
Median Wait Time	8 days
Delays	21 hours –14.6 days

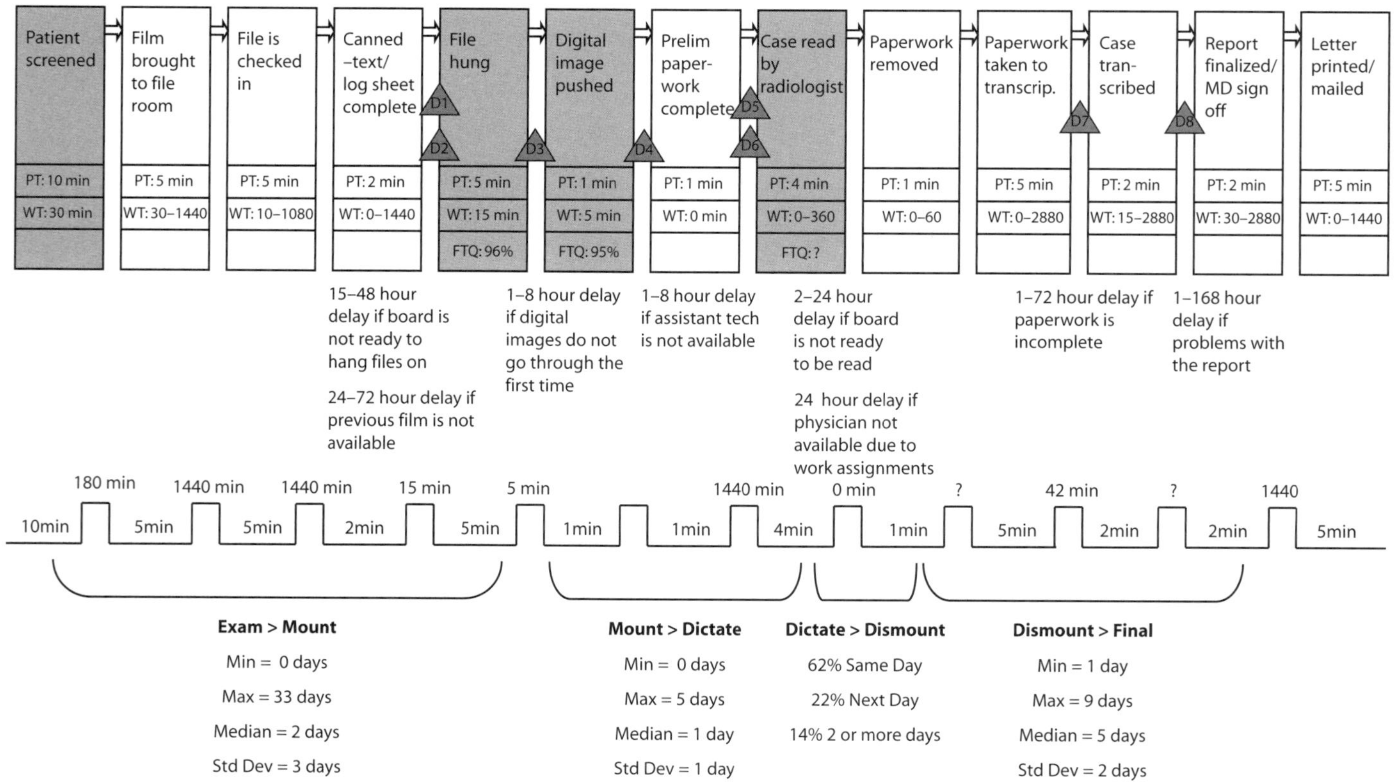

Figure 13.8(a) Current State Value Stream Map: Result Turnaround

Total Process Time	35 min
Value Added Time	18 min
Wait Time Range	30 min–28.5 hours
Median Wait Time	14.5 hours
Delays	?

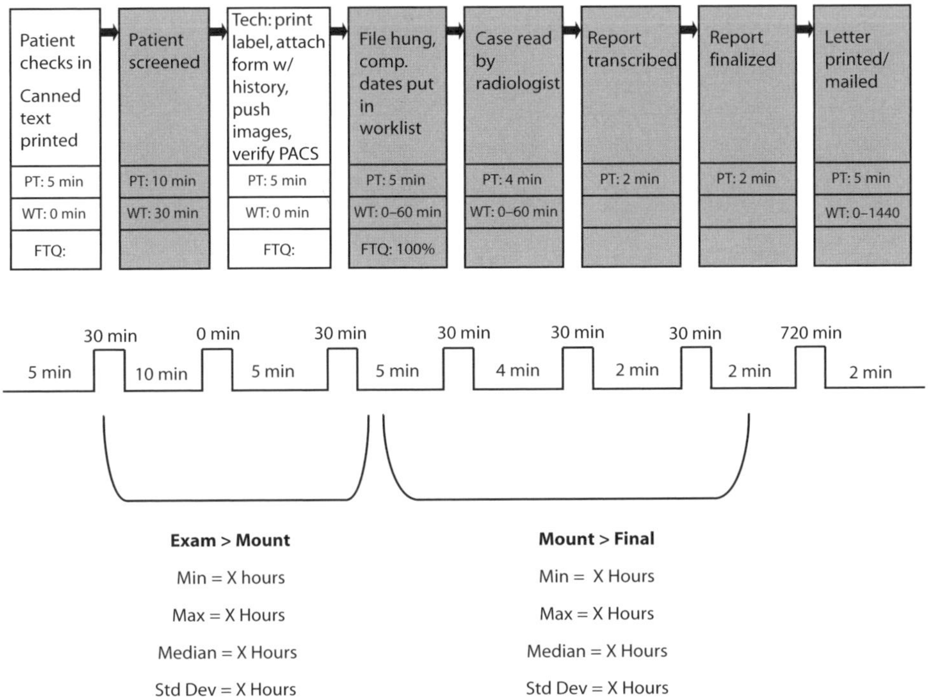

Figure 13.8(b) Future State Value Stream Map: Result Turnaround

3. Create a "current state" value stream map to depict the process as it is actually carried out, not as it is supposed to be.
4. If necessary, collect additional data, add them to the value stream map, and analyze the map to identify high priority areas of improvement to achieve goals.
5. Create a "future state" value stream map depicting the ideal process once any improvement activities are carried out.
6. Create a master action plan and carry out projects using Lean strategies or Six Sigma tools.

The Lean Strategies

As with Six Sigma and TQM, the Lean model includes a number of specific techniques and tools, such as SMED/Quick Changeover, total productive maintenance (TPM), mistake proofing, Just-in-Time (as described under TQM), and the five S's. Lean strategies encourage employees to look everywhere for waste and inefficiency and to think creatively for ways to eliminate them. Using techniques based on these strategies, for example, a Minneapolis ambulatory clinic was able to eliminate multiple waiting rooms and shorten patient waiting times by scheduling based on continuous flow (ie, appointments for the nurse, physician, and diagnostic testing were scheduled in sequence).[4] In Boston, a major medical center shortened wait times and improved imaging technologist efficiency by having patients self-check into an X-ray waiting area and signal electronically that they had arrived.[8]

Single Minute Exchange of Die/Quick Changeover

Single Minute Exchange of Die (SMED) is an approach to reducing output and quality losses due to changeovers. It's a technique used to analyze and reduce resources needed for equipment setup. For example, imaging facilities struggle with how to reduce wait times and costs for MRI patients.[20] The first solution may be to buy more equipment, which includes expensive MRI equipment. This solution, on the surface, seems to be appropriate and is the easiest and fastest—or is it? In planning for new equipment, more space, more trained people to operate the equipment, and more supplies are needed; the result is that the initial cost of buying the equipment was only the tip of the iceberg. The real solution should have been to analyze the entire process from the time patients arrive for their MRIs to the point they leave and determine how much time and activities are "waste." When this is done, much of the time is classified as waste and one of the wastes is the set-up time inbetween each patient.

Total Productive Maintenance

Total productive maintenance (TPM) is a program concept that brings maintenance into focus in order to minimize downtimes and maximize equipment usage. The three main goals of TPM are: zero breakdowns, zero defects, and zero accidents (eg, avoiding emergency repairs and keeping unscheduled maintenance to a minimum).

Mistake Proofing

Also called *Poka Yoke* (a Japanese term literally translated as "mistake proofing"), mistake proofing is a structured approach to ensure a quality and error-free environment. It incorporates simple mechanisms that either prevent errors from occurring or make errors obvious before serious consequences result. With the ACR's National Patient Safety Goals at the forefront of organizational operations, this technique is especially relevant. Incorporating processes to match patient and procedure materials (eg, bar coding), ensuring relevant information is available (eg, scripting), and moving information accurately through space and time (eg, via electronic medical and health records) would be associated with this technique.

The Five S's

This technique is considered critical to the implementation of all other improvement efforts. It's a common-sense tool, consisting of five steps used to carry out specific improvements as identified through value stream mapping[4]:

1. Sort: Supplies and small equipment should be sorted and only those items needed frequently should be kept in the immediate work area.
2. Shine: The workplace should be kept clean and equipment should be routinely maintained.
3. Straighten: Equipment and supplies should be arranged efficiently, based on the value stream map.
4. Systemize: Work processes should be governed by standards that are monitored and maintained.
5. Sustain: Audits, monitoring, and other systems, along with trained personnel, should be in place to ensure quality and performance gains achieved by applying the first four steps are maintained.

The five S's strategies significantly help both implement and sustain improvements. The gold standard for the five S's is that anyone should be able to find anything in their own workplace in less than 30 seconds, and anywhere else in the workplace in less than 5 minutes without talking to anyone, opening a book, or turning on a computer.[21]

To begin, first observe the process and create a spaghetti diagram. This is a map of the process including tasks done in sequence, location of supplies and equipment, distance traveled, and locations where time is wasted searching or waiting. Start by either printing out or drawing a diagram of the floor plan of the area that contains the process under evaluation. Identify the object/person to be tracked and its starting point on the map. Start the line and replicate the actual flow of the object/person on the map and continue the line until the completion of the process. The resulting line will most likely look like a piece of spaghetti, which is the source of its name. Visualizing the process in this manner will help find ways to change the sequence in which tasks are done or move supplies or equipment closer to where they're needed.

See Sidebar 13.2 for a case study on the five S's.

SIDEBAR 13.2: Case Study: Five S's

Problem: Chronically disorganized supply storerooms in the clinical laboratory at a medical facility contained critical documents, patient personal care items, and room conversion accessories, but did not provide adequate space for daily-use and must-have inventory supplies.

Symptoms:

- Supplies could not be located quickly, which led to reorder requisitions for items that were in stock but couldn't be found.
- Conducting inventories and ordering supplies took an excessive amount of time, reducing patient-service activities.
- Supply quantities varied widely with too many of some supplies and too little of others.
- Supply storerooms contained obsolete and expired items, leading to a false sense of having adequate supply quantities.
- It was found that staff horded supplies in personal areas because "they needed them" and "[the supply rooms] never have what I need," which skewed balances and monthly budget reviews.
- Staff complained that they needed more space.

Solution: The five S's team worked in two storerooms and achieved substantial progress in eliminating the problems. Storeroom improvements have been a great benefit to staff members and resulted in contracting for formal improvements using Lean Enterprise tools and principals. After the reorganization of the first storeroom, several individuals from the medical facility's anatomic pathology department were given a tour of the completed storeroom. When they saw what the team had achieved, they immediately requested the team's assistance and expertise in producing similar results in their storeroom. The five S's team replicated their success in the department storeroom and freed up 40% of the storeroom space by implementing methods similar to those they deployed in the clinical lab.

The project objective of improving ease of use was a resounding success. Staff can now ask colleagues who have never even seen the storeroom to retrieve an item, which can be located within 30 seconds.

Actions:

- Items were rearranged and segmented based on use.
- A "One-Point Lesson" poster, a visual prompt of how to quickly locate supply items, was placed in the supply room.
- An alphabetical list of all supply items was placed in the supply room doorway.
- The supply delivery schedule was changed from one large shipment per week to two smaller shipments that were easier to receive and place in stock.

Impact:

- A 17% increase in available storage space in the clinical lab storeroom was realized.
- Storage space in the anatomic pathology storeroom saw a 40% increase in storage space.
- Locations were reorganized resulting in staff ability to locate items within 30 seconds.
- Shipment frequency was doubled, decreasing the wait time for resupply without increasing costs.

Source: Adapted from Profero, Inc. Medical Storeroom Organization – 5S. Available at: http://www.lean.org/FuseTalk/Forum/Attachments/Case%20Study%20-%20Storeroom%20Organization%20-%205S.pdf. Accessed February 24, 2010.

Malcolm Baldrige National Quality Award

In 1987 the US Department of Commerce created the Malcolm Baldrige National Quality Award to enhance the competitiveness of the United States in the global economy. By recognizing achievements in quality and improved performance, the award also educates American businesses about the importance of quality as a competitive advantage. While the initial focus of the award program was manufacturing and service organizations, healthcare and education were eventually added as categories, with the first Malcolm Baldrige healthcare award granted in 2003.

The Baldrige Health Care Criteria for Performance Excellence can be a valuable resource for imaging facilities to evaluate their CQI efforts, no matter which quality model(s) the facility chooses to implement. The criteria are available free of charge from the National Institute of Standards and Technology. Even if a healthcare organization does not want to apply for the award, the published criteria can serve as a standard of measurement and a roadmap for further improvement.

The Baldrige performance excellence criteria include[22]:

- Leadership—how senior executives guide the organization and how the organization addresses its responsibilities to the public and practices good citizenship
- Strategic planning—how the organization sets strategic directions and determines key action plans
- Customer and market focus—how the organization determines requirements and expectations of customers and markets; builds relationships with customers; and acquires, satisfies, and retains customers
- Measurement, analysis, and knowledge management—the management, effective use, analysis, and improvement of data and information to support key processes and the organization's performance management system
- Human resource focus—how the organization enables its workforce to develop its full potential and how the workforce is aligned with the organization's objectives
- Process management—how key production/delivery and support processes are designed, managed, and improved
- Business results—the organization's performance and improvement in its key business areas: customer satisfaction, financial and marketplace performance, human resources, supplier and partner performance, operational performance, and governance and social responsibility, as well as how the organization performs relative to its competitors

The correspondence of the Baldrige criteria to imaging operations is apparent and relevant in either a freestanding imaging center or hospital-based setting. The key to accomplishing goals based on the above criteria is to gain facility-wide involvement and to be prepared to make incremental and, in some cases, substantial changes to the way business is done.

Leadership

Leadership may be the most difficult of the core concepts to implement. The others, however, cannot be accomplished without leadership and high-level organizational support (administrative leaders as well as radiologists) who must clearly communicate and demonstrate their commitment to a culture of process improvement and change.

Most employees, at some time or another in their work life, have encountered a "quality drive" that has fallen flat. Such failures can often be traced to the leadership's commitment to support and maintain the initiatives. It is difficult to maintain staff motivation for quality when management appears too distracted with the day-to-day running of the operation to attend to the quality program.

Employees will see through an underdeveloped attempt at leadership if they are blamed for errors and poor quality or have a fear of retribution, rather than working in an environment of collaboration and shared responsibility and accountability. In many organizations, developing an environment of continuous improvement and consistent quality calls for successfully implementing cultural change. Those in leadership roles must communicate the "why" of changes, consistently reinforce that message, and acknowledge that many employees will experience great difficulty embracing the instability and ambiguity that comes from change.

The first step in providing leadership for an organization is to set clear goals, with the assistance of those doing the work, and to eliminate the roadblocks to achieving those goals. Leaders have to lead but cannot "muscle through" the process; employee ownership and participation are musts in order to foster cooperation and the willingness to examine, change, and measure performance.

Encouraging participation from the people doing the work is true leadership. While not every idea is necessarily effective or feasible, the free flow of ideas shows respect and encourages flexibility and receptivity to change.

Strategic Planning

The effective, high-quality organization will be able to translate its strategic direction into a defined action plan and from this, to determine where process improvement is most needed in order to accomplish its business goals. Healthcare in general and imaging in particular function in a world in which external environmental factors are constantly changing, including how imaging services will be paid for and delivered.

A long-range outlook is a forward-thinking concept in that the organization has to commit to being a quality operation over time. The only way to ensure this is to be willing to accept industry changes while adapting the quality program to absorb those changes. Keeping an open mind and creating an environment that is comfortable with change makes a long-range outlook possible.

Customer and Market Focus

As noted before, a customer focus is characteristic of all CQI models, so it is not surprising that it comprises a Baldrige criterion. Whether those customers are internal (eg, a coworker) or external (eg, referring physicians), meeting and exceeding their needs and expectations drive process changes. Systems must be in place to measure and monitor satisfaction, to analyze data, and to initiate changes that will correct any deficiencies.

Measurement, Analysis, and Knowledge Management

No quality initiative is possible without effective and efficient data collection, analysis, and management, a fact acknowledged by the Baldrige criteria. Twenty-first-century technological developments can put massive amounts of data at an imaging administrator's fingertips, but the information is worthless without careful analysis and use. Systems must be in place and staff must be trained to identify what data need to be collected and how to put them to use to meet customer needs. The costs are high to install an imaging information system, PACS, electronic medical record system, and/or practice management system, but the costs of not doing so are even higher.

Human Resource Focus

Quality organizations recognize that their employees are one of their most valuable assets and put systems in place to effectively hire, coach, train, and develop each staff person to the best of his or her ability. The employees care for the customers and, as a result, will play a major role in determining customer satisfaction. In addition, facilities with a CQI focus recognize that employees are themselves internal customers whose needs must be met; doing so brings significant benefits. A Florida hospital that has won the Baldrige Award, for example, found its employee turnover was cut in half during the first 5 years of its quality efforts, and the hospital was designated one of the top 100 companies to work for by *Fortune* magazine.[23]

Process Management

In the CQI organization, the adage "If it's not broken, don't fix it" may be more appropriately worded "If it's not broken ... break it."

Change occurs rapidly in modern healthcare and more so in imaging. With rapid-fire developments in both information and technology—clinical and managerial—some organizations may suddenly realize they are still utilizing outdated support processes that were in place before new technology solutions were implemented and operational workflow dramatically altered as a result. Quality facilities have systems in place to monitor and anticipate process obsolescence. They acknowledge that "we've always done it that way" is not a reason for continuing a process that no longer meets customer needs. These organizations solicit employee suggestions, analyze customer data, review flow charts and other quality tools, and when problems are identified, use their CQI model to improve. One Baldrige healthcare winner, for example, generated 6800 suggestions for process changes and implemented 5000 of them in a single year.[23]

With true process improvement, the root cause of the problem may lay several layers away from the problem's manifestation. Therefore, a team represented by several departments may be the best way to find a solution to the cause of the problem. This type of problem solving helps to avoid a cursory "fix" to what may or may not be the actual problem.

Business Results

The Baldrige criteria recognize that high quality and solid business results are linked. As with the CQI models themselves, the award emphasizes the need for ongoing measurements of a range of business parameters, acknowledging the wisdom of the precept "You can't manage what you can't measure." In particular, the quality criteria recognize the importance of establishing and achieving measurable goals in the following areas to bring about better than average business results:

1. Customer satisfaction: Quality organizations rely on surveys, focus groups, and other tools to measure and monitor satisfaction of all their internal and external customers; use the data collected to guide improvement efforts; and reinforce the customer focus at every level of the business.
2. Financial and marketplace performance: Sound financial practice enables facilities to invest in quality measures, technological advancements, and employee development. Important performance measures include determination of market share, comparison with competitors, and improvements in financial performance (ie, gains in business as well as reductions in operational overhead).

3. Human resources: Quality cannot be achieved without qualified, motivated employees, so human resource goals must be set for hiring to promote quality; measuring and maintaining employee satisfaction; rewarding desired behaviors and job performance; and providing skill-based training/education.
4. Supplier and partner performance: Recognizing that quality is not achieved in a vacuum, organizations must put procedures in place to ensure vendors also meet quality expectations and to build a "partnership" relationship with vendors and service providers.
5. Operational performance: The organization must have procedures in place that guide how business processes are selected, analyzed, and measured for improvement results.
6. Governance and social responsibility: Quality organizations have established policies and procedures to measure and maintain effective governance, and they demonstrate social responsibility within their profession and community.

Conclusion

A range of CQI tools is available for performance improvement in an imaging facility. The key is to find an accessible method that fits the organization's goals, can be supported by practice data, and has the full commitment of senior management. Buy in from radiologists, administrators, and supervisors is essential for the success of any quality improvement program, which should not be viewed as a quick fix but rather a long-term effort that the organization is dedicated to seeing through. In such a highly regulated and competitive field, a facility committed to CQI may very well emerge as an industry leader.

References

1. Agency for Healthcare Research and Quality, U.S. Department of Health and Human Services. Your guide to choosing quality healthcare: a quick look at quality. Available at: http://www.ahrq.gov/consumer/qnt/qntqlook.htm. Accessed May 15, 2009.

2. Savage GT, Williams ES. Performance improvement in health care: the quest to achieve quality. In: Buchbinder SB, Shanks NH, eds. *Introduction to Health Care Management*. Boston, MA: Jones and Bartlett; 2007: 81–135.

3. Griffith JR, White KR. *The Well-Managed Healthcare Organization*. 5th ed. Washington, DC: AUPHA Press; 2002.

4. Varkey P, Reller MK, Resar RK. Basics of quality improvement in health care. *Mayo Clin Proc*. 2007;82:735–739.

5. Hashmi K. Introduction and implementation of Total Quality Management (TQM). *iSixSigma.com.* Available at: http://www.isixsigma.com/index.php?option=com_k2&view=item&id=1489:introduction-and-implementation-of-total-quality-management-tqm&Itemid=179 Accessed March 23, 2010.

6. Goetsch DL, Davis SB. *Introduction to Total Quality: Quality Management for Production, Processing and Services.* Englewood Cliffs, NJ: Prentice-Hall; 1997.

7. Capezio P, Morehouse D. *Taking the Mystery Out of TQM: A Practical Guide to Total Quality Management.* 2nd ed. Franklin Lakes, NJ: Career Press; 1995.

8. Loria K. Go lean: lean manufacturing. *DOTmed News.* Available at: http://www.dotmed.com/dm7993. Published March 4, 2009. Accessed April 22, 2009.

9. Gonzalez CM, Jang T, Raines M, Lys TZ, Schaeffer AJ. Significant clinical practice cost savings through downsizing office supply inventory and just in time ordering. *J Urol.* 2006;176:267–269.

10. Harry M, Schroeder R. *Six Sigma.* New York, NY: Currency/Doubleday; 2000.

11. Bounds G, Yorks L, Adams M, Ranney G. *Beyond Total Quality Management: Toward the Emerging Paradigm.* New York, NY: McGraw-Hill; 1994.

12. Scalise D. Six Sigma: the quest for quality. *Hosp Health Networks.* 2001;75(12):41–45.

13. Cherry J, Seshadri S. Six Sigma: using statistics to reduce process variability and costs in radiology. *Radiol Manage.* 2000;22(6):42–45.

14. Viau M, Southern B. Six Sigma and Lean concepts, a case study: patient centered care model for a mammography center. *Radiol Manage.* 2007;29(5):19–28.

15. Benedetto AR. Six Sigma: not for the faint of heart. *Radiol Manage.* 2003;25(2):40–53.

16. Endsley S, Magill MK, Godfrey MM. Creating a lean practice. *Fam Pract Manag.* 2006;13(4):34–38.

17. Bertels T. Integrating Lean and Six Sigma. *iSixSigma.com.* Available at: http://www.isixsigma.com/index.php?option=com_k2&view=item&id=1386&Itemid=156. Accessed March 23, 2010.

18. iSixSigma. Quality dictionary and glossary. Available at: http://www.isixsigma.com/dictionary/Value_Stream_Mapping-413.htm. Accessed February 24, 2010.

19. Haas R, Torgerson C. Value stream mapping in a patient care unit. Society for Health Systems Archived Webcast. Available at: http://www.shsweb.org/webcasts/valueStream.htm. Accessed May 11, 2009.

20. KAIZEN Institute Lean Advisors. SMED/Quick Changeover—the payoff. Available at: http://www.leanadvisors.com/index.php/impact/articles_full/smed_quick_changeover_the_payoff/. Accessed February 24, 2010.

21. Skinner C. 5S: The Lean Roadmap. SAE International. Available at: http://www.sae.org/manufacturing/lean/column/leannov01.htm. Accessed February 24, 2010.

22. National Institute of Standards and Technology. Frequently asked questions about the Malcolm Baldrige National Quality Award. Available at: http://www.nist.gov/public_affairs/factsheet/baldfaqs.htm. Accessed May 15, 2009.

23. McLaughlin CP, Kaluzny AD, eds. *Continuous Quality Improvement in Health Care: Theory, Implementations, and Applications*. 3rd ed. Boston, MA: Jones and Bartlett; 2006.

Chapter 14

Develop a Quality Improvement Program

Jennifer Kroken

Successfully implementing a continuous quality improvement program is a highly challenging project. The issues affecting the probability of success are the strength of senior management's commitment to change, the availability of talented leadership and other resources, and effective improvement teams. Most organizations will find many more opportunities for quality improvement than there are resources; among the key areas to focus on are patient access, the patient experience, and report turnaround. Selection of the appropriate program relies on features of the quality models and factors related to the organization.

Too many healthcare organizations continue to operate believing that there is nothing in their processes that need improvement; they can remain competitive with the status quo; and mistakes are inevitable in a people-based service industry. Such thinking ignores the many published reports of hospitals and outpatient facilities that have eliminated life-threatening medical errors, saved thousands and even millions of dollars, and/or nurtured a customer focus.[1–3] Putting their own practices under the microscope, searching out the best practices of others, and implementing quality improvement models[4] made these success stories happen.

No one wants to make mistakes, cause patients harm, or waste time or money. Employees do not enjoy facing irate patients or vendors nor do they want to lose their jobs because their organizations failed to meet financial goals. Employees want to work for a successful organization that meets the needs of patients, referring physicians, vendors, and the community. An effective quality improvement program can help achieve that success.

Factors to Consider in the Choice of a Quality Improvement Model

At least four models are currently in use in healthcare facilities to achieve continuous quality improvement (CQI): Total Quality Management (TQM), FOCUS-PDCA, Six Sigma, and Lean. Some organizations may use a combination of models, while others base their quality improvement programs on the criteria of the

Baldrige National Quality Award or the standards of The Joint Commission. CQI is less about the model chosen and more about moving forward to meet customer needs and achieve desired outcomes.

Nevertheless, basing a program on a model or combination of models has its advantages. The specialized terminology and processes of the models help a facility's staff to distinguish the effort from either prior experience (with less successful predecessors) or the status quo. Testing of the methodologies has identified best practices, eliminating trial and error. If a consultant or in-house expert is hired to lead the effort, using an existing model provides a basis for understanding expectations and common ground from which to carry out the facility-specific program.

Managerial Factors

A healthcare organization planning to implement a CQI program has several options with regard to personnel to manage and lead the program:

1. One or more current employees can be trained in the specific methodologies and, in turn, will train other employees as appropriate. Depending on the size of the organization, available funds, and the model selected, the quality leader may take on the CQI duties in addition to his or her regular assignment.
2. A new staff member can be hired whose job is to manage the CQI effort, a so-called in-house expert or internal consultant. This senior level manager should have experience in several of the models and be accountable for the success of the program and for directing staff members who carry out individual projects in addition to their regular assignments.
3. An experienced independent contractor can be hired for a defined period to lead the effort and train employees to eventually assume leadership. This individual is likely to have experience in a particular model, so the organization may need to choose its preferred methodology before issuing a request for proposal.
4. A quality management consulting firm can be hired to provide services similar to those of the independent contractor. The firm may offer a broader range of experience and resources, but may lack the full-time commitment of an independent contractor.

These options comprise what Six Sigma consultant Edoardo Monopoli has called "the buy-make-rent dilemma." He suggests the following factors should influence the choice of option[5]:

- Value—To what extent does the position (and the quality program) impact the facility's strategic success? A major effort, such as Six Sigma or Total Quality Management, is likely to be crucial to this success.

- Uniqueness—How readily available are the needed skills in the labor market? How unique is the facility's culture, which may make understanding it or working with staff difficult for an outsider?

If the value placed on the effort is high and the culture of the organization is unique, an organization would be best served by developing its own experts internally. If strategic value is low and uniqueness not a factor, using an independent contractor at least initially may make the most sense. If the strategic value is high and the labor market offers a number of experienced individuals (low uniqueness), then hiring a full-time quality leader is the best solution. Finally, when the facility's quality program is not viewed as strategically vital (often the case when a program first starts), but the uniqueness factor is high, contracting with a consulting firm will allow the program to achieve some results quickly.

Model Factors

Three activities comprise the core of all CQI models[4]:

- Collecting and evaluating data related to current operations
- Involving staff in all phases, from problem identification to implementation of solutions
- Continuously seeking new and innovative opportunities to improve

While the fundamentals may be similar, the differences in the models make some more suitable for certain organizations or problems than for others. The models can be divided into two categories, evolutionary and revolutionary.[6] Evolutionary methods, including TQM, FOCUS-PDCA, and Lean, are best applied to relatively minor problems for which modest incremental improvements are sought. These methods do not involve major process redesign, and they are less disruptive in the workplace. Revolutionary methods, with Six Sigma being the most commonly applied example in healthcare, are needed when problems cross departmental boundaries or call for drastic measures. Revolutionary methods may also be useful when merging two practices that do not share common procedures or technology or are geographically dispersed. Table 14.1 compares other factors that may influence the selection process.

Organizational Factors

A study of primary care medical groups identified a number of factors that were most valuable in their success in improving quality.[7] These factors were grouped into five categories, the most important of which were the organizational capability for change and an infrastructure for implementation. Specifically, the experienced physicians and coordinators who led the quality projects ranked the organizational factors in Box 14.1 as the 21 most important.

Table 14.1 Differences Between Six Sigma and Evolutionary CQI Models

Characteristic	*Six Sigma*	*Evolutionary*
Degree of improvement sought	>20%	<20%
Approach	Statistically based problem solving	Various, eg, best practices, value stream mapping
Length of projects	12–24 months	Weeks
Number of simultaneous projects per department	One	Several
Scope	Interdepartmental or institutional	Intradepartmental or institutional
Impact on personnel	Probable job restructuring; staffing increases or decreases	Changes in work processes; isolated impact on staffing
Training	Multiple sessions focused on the five steps, with real-world application between each	Short workshops on key principles with real-world application between each

Evolutionary models include Total Quality Management, FOCUS-PCDA, and Lean.

Sources: Benedetto AR. Six Sigma: not for the faint of heart. *Radiol Manage*. 2003;25(2):40–53. Bertels T. Integrating Lean and Six Sigma: the power of an integrated roadmap. *iSixSigma.com*. Available at: http://www.isixsigma.com/library/content/c030721a.asp. Accessed March 23, 2010.

Box 14.1 Most Valuable Factors in Achieving Quality (in descending order of importance)

1. Presence of organized systems in the practice
2. Commitment to change by the leadership
3. Project leadership by enthusiastic volunteers
4. Internal clinician champions for clinical guideline projects
5. Priorities for quality versus financial by the group
6. Resources available for implementation
7. CQI understanding and skills
8. Collaborative working environment
9. Clinician cohesiveness to shared mission and policies
10. Relative advantage that accrues from the new process
11. Importance to clinicians of the new guideline topic
12. Standardized organizational process for making change
13. Change management infrastructure well developed
14. Internal clinician interest in making the changes
15. Internal turmoil present from internal status quo
16. Leadership support for steps to fulfill the vision
17. Management authorization of resources for project
18. Strategic plan inclusion of implementation in annual goals
19. Resource agreement process in place at all organizational levels
20. Active leadership involvement personally in the change process
21. Organizational culture supportive of the planned change(s)

Source: Solberg LI, Kottke TE, Brekke. Quality improvement in primary care: the role of organization, collaboratives, and managed care. In: McLaughlin CP, Kaluzny AD, eds. *Continuous Quality Improvement in Health Care: Theory, Implementations, and Applications*. 3rd ed. Boston, MA: Jones and Bartlett; 2006.

Organizations that believe Six Sigma will be the most appropriate model for the problems being addressed should evaluate themselves on additional factors. First, Six Sigma's heavy reliance on data-based decision making is poorly matched to circumstances in which personalities (eg, the physician with the highest billings) or politics (institutional or governmental) drive decisions. Second, to achieve the necessary level of change, Six Sigma may result in job restructuring, staff reductions or increases, or changes in stakeholder relationships; the organization's leaders must be willing to consider *all* options and make unpopular decisions, as circumstances dictate. Third, if the imaging service is part of a larger institution (eg, a hospital-based imaging department), a problem warranting Six Sigma will likely require participation by other departments. The departmental leadership, as well as the institution's senior management, must perceive value in the project, understand the model, and be willing to commit to major changes.

Priorities to Consider in Choice of Process to Improve

No matter how well a facility operates, the likelihood is that many opportunities exist for quality improvement. The first step of any CQI initiative is to identify one or more processes as potentially benefiting from changes. Faced with data analyzed via Pareto charts, scatter diagrams, flowcharts, and other tools, the CQI team may still find more opportunities than there are resources available. Applying additional criteria may help narrow the focus.

In the case of clinical processes, four categories of information may be useful[8]:

1. Data related to patient care, such as adverse effects, negative outcomes, incidents, complaints, and malpractice claims: Problems in these areas can have a high cost in terms of both quality and finances; thus, improvements can have a relatively high impact on the organization. Trends away from benchmarks signal areas that should be examined further.
2. Data from satisfaction surveys of patients, families, referring physicians, and other customers: Negative changes in responses to key questions over time, as well as specific participant comments, may indicate areas that need a closer examination.
3. Financial data, especially related to the total cost per patient or per examination: Faced with increased pressure to control costs, facilities with higher than industry-average costs may be confronted with hard choices. While lower costs are not guaranteed to result from all CQI projects, efforts that improve productivity and efficiency and reduce waste will boost the bottom line over time.

4. Changes in clinical practice guidelines: Implementing new guidelines from professional or accrediting organizations may necessitate changes in multiple processes or patient care areas. This is an ideal opportunity to examine these processes and make other changes that will improve overall quality.

In the case of nonclinical processes, five additional considerations may be useful:

1. Strategic objectives: Target customer satisfaction, market share, and financial performance processes that contribute directly to the organization's strategic objectives.
2. High gains for a modest outlay: Improve processes that consume significant resources or that have a high cost of quality.
3. Short turnaround time: Improvements can likely be carried out within a short timeframe, or a process that has a relatively short (3 months or less) cycle time from input to output.
4. Satisfaction: The current process is highly disruptive and the improvement of which will boost staff morale.
5. Manageability: The process is not too complex or broad; its improvement will not require more resources than are available.

Applying these criteria to the three operational areas that are particularly important to patients and referring physicians—patient access, the patient experience, and report turnaround—can provide a solid basis for an effective CQI program (Sidebar 14.1).

Identifying Issues of Patient Access

Patient access to imaging services is a fundamental aspect of care for patients, referring physicians, and health insurance plans. From the customer's perspective, responsibility for prompt access falls primarily on the front desk staff and secondarily on the technologists to move patients quickly through the department. However, many factors "behind the scenes" can either enhance or detract from accessibility and must be taken into account in CQI efforts.

If problems with patient access are revealed through customer surveys, analysis of throughput data, and staff suggestions, the CQI team will need to assess both staff functioning and behind-the-scenes factors. One is equipment availability. Is the schedule full? If not, are certain modalities obviously lagging behind others in capacities? If the facility is multimodal but has only one machine per modality, the technologist's efficiency is crucial, but so is equipment function (or malfunction). Most scheduling software allows for blocks of time to be reserved for each machine. The improvement assessment will need to make sure an appropriate amount of

SIDEBAR 14.1: Case Study: One Facility's Success with Six Sigma

At the start of the project, a Florida hospital-based women's breast center conducted over 42,000 procedures annually. However, its no-show rate for follow-up appointments by women with suspicious findings on their initial screening mammography was about 30%. These patients were going elsewhere because of lengthy waits for appointments, averaging 13 weeks from first appointment for screening to biopsy results.

The team set a target goal of reducing the process to 4 weeks, with a stretch goal of no more than 2 weeks. The first step was to analyze the current process, revealing significant variation. A value stream map and priority matrix identified three key areas with the greatest potential for improvement: before the appointment, during the appointment, and after the appointment. Teams were formed to address each one.

The next step sought to streamline the patient experience by completely redesigning the diagnostic workflow during the appointments. The most important development was facilitating all of the patient's pre-biopsy diagnostic work to be done in one appointment, including the screening mammography, a diagnostic mammography, and breast ultrasound. On the same day, she could meet with the reviewing radiologist and the nurse educator for additional information and to make an appointment for breast biopsy and possibly a breast MRI examination.

The process resulted in reducing the average turnaround time to 3 weeks for delivery of biopsy results. In addition, 10% more appointment slots were created and the need for an additional digital mammography unit was justified through Six Sigma data analysis.

Source: Viau M, Southern B. Six Sigma and Lean concepts, a case study: patient centered care model for a mammography center. *Radiol Manage*. 2007;29(5):19–28.

time is blocked for each modality. The team will also need to review equipment operational records and agreements with vendors that provide for minimal downtime and replacement equipment.

A flowchart of the patient scheduling process may reveal elements in need of improvement. If the frontline staff's goal is to keep the referring physician's staff on the telephone for as short a time as possible, is the information they collect adequate but not excessive? For example, is enough information collected so staff can determine if prior authorization is needed?

The quality improvement team may also need to analyze the facility's hours of operation. What is the earliest date/time a patient can get in for an examination? Does the facility accommodate walk-ins? Anecdotally, does it continually close later than the established closing hours?

The radiologist's availability is also a factor in patient access. Ideally, a radiologist is onsite for the entire workday, but many facilities have to share radiologists. In such instances, scheduling takes on another dimension to ensure examinations requiring the presence of a radiologist (eg, those with contrast) are scheduled on the appropriate days.

Identifying Issues Related to the Patient Experience

The patient experience actually begins with the scheduling process, before he or she ever enters the facility. Assuming the group has achieved success with regard to access, the patient experience continues with the patient walking through the door, being greeted in reception, waiting, undergoing the procedure, and receiving the test results. Thus, the experience is comprised of a series of processes, involving nearly all of the facility's staff, and offering numerous opportunities for CQI. Among the areas calling for close scrutiny by the improvement team are patient check-in, transfer to the procedure area, and administration of the procedure.

- **Patient check-in:** Observation, flowcharting, patient surveys, and reception staff suggestions may reveal improvement projects to enhance this portion of the patient experience. To lessen patient anxiety, the reception area should offer a comfortable, calming environment; the staff should demonstrate competence, with a calm and welcoming demeanor. Procedures should be in place to elicit any necessary patient information in confidence and with minimal distractions. Contingency plans should allow staff to handle problems in a well-organized manner (eg, if the patient arrives without test orders or equipment is inoperable).
- **Transfer to the procedure area:** The procedure is the focal point of a patient's visit, unless obstacles interfere with the smooth transition from waiting room to procedure room. Once again, a flowchart can be a useful tool to identify factors that can result in patients spending too much time in the reception area, waiting too long in the procedure room before a technologist begins the procedure, or experiencing confusion or uncertainty because of inadequate instructions.
- **The procedure:** The responsibility for this portion of the patient's visit lies squarely on the shoulders of the technologists, so their input on possible improvements is essential. Patient satisfaction data will also be particularly helpful in identifying CQI projects for this part of the patient experience. For example, patients will often experience greater anxiety and be less satisfied if they are uncertain about what to expect from the procedure. Thus, technologists should be trained to consistently explain key elements: how long the procedure will take, if it will be painful or uncomfortable, and when the results will be available.

The technologist should also be able to confidently answer any additional questions or address any concerns. Furthermore, although the technologist is tasked with keeping the schedule moving, patients will enjoy their experience more if they do not feel rushed or as if they are an imposition.

The AIDET Philosophy

AIDET is a communication tool that lends consistency to interactions with patients and each other. It is an acronym of Acknowledgement, Introduction, Duration, Explanation, Thank you that represents a very powerful way to communicate with patients who are often nervous, anxious, and feeling vulnerable. When interacting with patients, gaining trust is essential for obtaining patient compliance and improving clinical outcomes. AIDET provides a consistent framework for staff to communicate with patients and families as well as each other. Below is an example of how it works[9]:

- A—Acknowledge the patient by greeting them with a smile: "Good morning, Mr. Brown. It's good to see you today."
- I—Introduce yourself and tell patients about your experience and background: "Hi, I'm Dr. Meacham. I'll be caring for you today. I thought it would help you if I gave you a little background information on me. I graduated from the University of Colorado, Denver. I have been in practice for 20 years and at UCD for 15 years."
- D—Duration: Tell the patient how long your part of their care will take and the approximate time before the next caregiver will see them. "This procedure will take about 15 minutes; and you will recover for about another 15 minutes."
- E—Explain the process "Here's what you can expect in your visit today: We are going to..."
- T—Thank the patient and make it personal: "Thanks, Mr. Jones, for visiting with us today. If you have questions after this visit, please call and ask for my nurse, Jenny, she will be able to answer them for you. She will confer with me as needed."

See Sidebar 14.2 for implementation guidelines, with the goals being for all staff to learn steps and benefits of AIDET and to achieve staff competency of AIDET skills.

Identifying Issues of Report Turnaround

Timely delivery of results to the referring physician and thereby to the patient is characteristic of quality-driven organizations; report turnaround can separate a good facility from an outstanding one. Referring physicians count on the results to

SIDEBAR 14.2: Sample Implementation Plan for AIDET

TIMELINE

Month 1:
Develop AIDET game plan and roll out to leaders and have leaders begin acting as role models.

Months 2 and 3:
Roll out AIDET to staff and post communication posters/flyers.

Month 4:
Have each department develop a competency checklist.

Months 5 and 6:
Taking the Introduction to a new level.

- Have departments share with one another their training, experience, what they do, and their technology.
- Create bio cards so that staff can learn about other staff's training in their department.

Months 7 and 8:
Expanding on time and procedures.

- Teams develop time expectation cards for different areas (eg, emergency department would set time expectations on test turnaround time).

Month 9:
Expanding on Thank You Notes

- Implement patient thank you cards from staff.

Source: Adapted from Studer Group. AIDET^{SM} Five Fundamentals of Patient Communication. 2005. Available at: http://www.studergroup.com/store/contentlet/AIDETImplementationTool1.pdf. Accessed March 23, 2010.

guide the patient's care; delays can negatively affect not only the patient's health but also the physician–patient relationship. Expectations are high: With the proliferation of PACS and voice-activated dictation, report turnaround should be easier to accomplish than it was a decade ago. Systems are available that allow referring physicians to see when the examination was completed, starting the clock for the radiologist to complete the report and send it to the referring physician promptly.

Focus groups, satisfaction surveys, or one-on-one interviews of referring physicians will be useful in revealing potential turnaround problems. An improvement team that includes at least one radiologist, along with administrative, clerical, and information technology (IT) staff, can follow up by analyzing data on report turnaround times using control charts, scatter diagrams, Pareto charts, and histograms. These and other CQI tools may reveal areas of improvement that relate to inconsistent work practices by radiologists, the need for technology upgrades, or process failures.

Preparing to Build a Successful CQI Program

There have been 10 rules identified for success in implementing TQM, which can be applied to any quality initiative[10]:

1. The chief executive officer must be committed to the program.
2. The reason(s) for the program must be clearly and consistently communicated to all stakeholders.
3. Senior managers must be committed to the program.
4. The organization must recognize the initiative as a team effort.
5. Leadership must be effective, participatory, and consistently committed.
6. No one aspect of the initiative should take precedence over the others (eg, TQM is about more than statistical process control).
7. Effort should be made, especially at the beginning, to work employees gradually into a major quality initiative.
8. Training is essential for all employees; some models require much more than others. It is important not to cut corners, while at the same time carrying out the training in a compressed fashion to keep momentum.
9. The quality initiative should be highly visible throughout the organization.
10. Accountability is the key to true culture change.

Sidebar 14.3 lists additional process improvement tips that can help ensure a successful quality program implementation.

Building Effective Quality Improvement Teams

Although the name and task(s) of teams may vary among the quality models, all models rely heavily on teams to move the program forward. Given their importance, an effort should be made to build and maintain effective teams.

Characteristics of Effective Teams

First, quality teams should have a clear idea of their task(s) and authority, which will vary with the project and organization. Is the team to be charged with identifying a problem, collecting data and analyzing it, evaluating possible solutions and making recommendations to senior management, implementing a solution, or all of the above? If a team's task includes implementation, are there constraints on the types of solutions that can be considered (eg, budgetary or staffing)? Does the team have the formal and informal authority necessary to impose the solution on affected staff?

SIDEBAR 14.3: Tips for Carrying Out a Successful CQI Program

- Focus on the process under review, not on people to blame for its shortcomings.
- Keep the goal of meeting the customers' needs uppermost.
- If the scope of a process is too broad, consider working on a component of the process.
- Improvement teams should include staff members who are involved with the process being analyzed and who are willing and able to be a voice to and from other staff.
- Resist the temptation to focus on solutions before analysis is complete and causes have been identified.
- Avoid skipping steps of the chosen model, but adapt techniques and tools when necessary.
- Process maps, control charts, and the other CQI tools are just that—tools. Avoid getting hung up on producing perfect charts.
- Once a process has been tested and the desired results obtained, create a new process map to help standardize the changes.
- Rely on facts and data, not assumptions and perceptions.
- Be creative; look for ways to innovate; challenge the status quo.
- Technology is not the solution to every problem; sometimes simple or "low-tech" solutions will achieve the desired results.
- Communication is essential and should be ongoing throughout the program.

Sources: Capezio P, Morehouse D. *Taking the Mystery Out of TQM: A Practical Guide to Total Quality Management*. 2nd ed. Franklin Lakes, NJ: Career Press; 1995: 317–318. Viau M, Southern B. Six Sigma and Lean concepts, a case study: patient centered care model for a mammography center. *Radiol Manage*. 2007;29(5):19–28.

Second, the team's size and composition should be appropriate for the task. Size needs to be large enough to include the necessary expertise but not so large that it becomes logistically difficult to schedule meetings and otherwise manage the group. Team members should represent all stakeholders who will affect or be directly affected by the team's decisions. This diversity will increase the likelihood that information crucial to identifying the problem or its solution(s) will be available within the team and that consensus for implementation can be reached before the solution is tested, thus decreasing potential opposition.

Third, no characteristic is likely to have greater impact on the team's effectiveness than the degree to which roles and relationships outside the team influence behavior and opinions within the team. Technologists who have less authority and status than radiologists may feel less willing to express their opinions or take on team roles that may put them at odds with the physician. In other cases, existing interpersonal problems or interprofessional rivalries may interfere with the team's function. To lessen the impact of these problems, the team leader should be someone with sufficient authority and respect among the various factions to effectively moderate behavior. The leader should be skilled at (1) ensuring lower status employees are not left out of the process and are encouraged to express opinions; (2) controlling higher status members, when necessary; and (3) defusing tension from hostile members.[11]

A related factor is the level of psychological safety team members feel within the group. Open and frank communication can only happen when all members believe they will not be condescended to or criticized for their comments. Members who feel unsafe will hesitate to take part in discussions and may express their opinions privately to "safe" colleagues, thus increasing the probability of failure for the initiative. An organization in which lower status employees are criticized for being negative when they express concerns on the job will have a difficult time creating a climate of psychological safety within the quality team. Members are likely to feel they will suffer repercussions outside the team for any opinions they may express. It may be necessary to address the lack of psychological safety in the workplace before starting the quality program.

Finally, the team norms should be recognized, consciously set, and reviewed as the need arises. Norms govern the standards of behavior and performance for team members. Behavioral norms incorporate elements such as meeting attendance, acceptable language, the use of formal procedures (eg, Robert's Rules of Order), and methods for reaching consensus and making decisions. Performance norms set expectations about the amount and quality of work to be performed by team members. Functional performance norms will help ensure that all team members know what is expected of them as they take on assignments, one team member does not carry the workload for the entire committee, and the team will meet assignment deadlines.

Basic Needs of Effective Teams

Quality improvement teams cannot function without adequate resources and support. Resources go beyond the financial ones to include member skills and knowledge, equipment, communication systems, information, and credibility. Providing these resources is one of the key ways senior management demonstrates its commitment to the quality initiative.

Teams and individual members also need to be recognized and rewarded for their project work. Recognition may be in the form of personal satisfaction when recommendations are implemented, a more efficient and pleasant working environment, or the feedback of coworkers and managers. Compensation should be given for meetings held after working hours or substantial project work carried out after hours. Rewards should be incorporated into the performance appraisal and given as incentive pay programs to acknowledge the effort involved beyond the employees' primary job description. (For more on reward and recognition systems, see another AHRA book, *Human Resource Management in Radiology*.)

Leaders are an important factor in the effectiveness of teams. A true leader is able to achieve the team's goals by influencing the members' behavior. Such leadership may arise informally from within the group or more formally by the appointment of a respected colleague. Because quality teams are largely problem-solving mechanisms, the leader's style must encourage participation, build trust, and support member risk taking with regard to expressing opinions. The leader must keep members engaged in the process, motivated to participate and carry out assignments, and stimulated to creativity and innovation. A major quality program will have multiple teams running consecutively and/or concurrently with different leaders, providing numerous opportunities for employees at various levels to demonstrate and hone their leadership skills.

Facing the Challenges

Implementing a program that will affect the entire organization, probably consume substantial resources, and disrupt work patterns (even temporarily) will present challenges that could derail the effort.

For example, most CQI models require substantial data to be collected and retained throughout the effort, which may produce IT challenges not immediately obvious to those starting a quality program. An imaging facility's computer system may work well for patient scheduling, but may not be able to provide adequate data on procedures. Historical data may not be available on a key metric, delaying the start of the project while baseline data can be collected. In the case of Six Sigma projects that continue for months or even a year or more, mechanisms must be in place that allow for consistent data collection, even if procedure codes change during the collection period. Some organizations may use different procedural definitions in different departments (eg, a combined chest and abdomen CT examination may count as one procedure for scheduling but two for productivity purposes). Before data collection can begin, all parties must create and agree on standardized definitions of procedures, as well as a way to identify and capture existing data using the new definitions. Furthermore, as personnel changes occur, new employees must be trained in data entry and collection processes; new supervisors must be shown how to monitor and audit these activities.

Changes in personnel can also have a negative impact on productivity. Valuable continuity is lost when the inevitable turnover occurs; new team members must be quickly appointed and brought up to date on progress. As the program continues, pressure may build for CQI team members to skip meetings or resign from the committee. From time to time, senior management may need to remind supervisors of the project's importance to the organization.

The program's length can have other consequences. Interest and enthusiasm may flag among team members and other stakeholders, especially during the lengthy Six Sigma projects. The leader must find ways to motivate participants and reignite interest, such as regular staff updates on even relatively small accomplishments or devising interim short-term goals to celebrate when achieved.

One of the factors affecting the length of the project may be the facility's IT capabilities. Data collection and analysis, simulations to test solutions, and form and/or process changes that are pilot tested and then implemented will probably all involve IT. One or more IT staff will need to be assigned to the project. The project manager will have to discuss specific needs with these IT professionals, who in turn will have to describe to the project manager what the process will be to meet those needs. Additional programming may need to occur, reports to be written, and software to be updated—all of which can be time consuming. As the CQI project continues, unanticipated system deficiencies may arise, slowing or even halting progress. If the facility uses outside vendors to provide its IT support, the entire process is likely to take even longer.

Those involved in initiating and managing the CQI program should also be prepared to deal with rumors about the motivation for and likely consequences of the effort. Any process that produces substantial change, uncertainty, and fear will lead to rumors. If untrue and left unaddressed, these can lessen participation and cooperation, lower morale, increase staff turnover, and lower customer quality. Leaders need to anticipate rumors and preempt them with public announcements; communicate truthfully and as fully as possible about projected outcomes; and provide opportunities for employees to ask questions and get information.

Conclusion

A number of factors go into operating a successful imaging facility, many of which relate to the satisfaction of the patients and referring physicians. That satisfaction is achieved when the patient's total experience is comprised of convenient scheduling, ease of check-in, short waiting times, an efficient but thorough procedure, and prompt communication with the referring physician. Creating and maintaining a quality program that delivers excellent service is predicated on meeting the needs of patients, physicians, and other customers of the organization.

CQI is an effective means to ensure that excellent service is delivered consistently, by using quality measurement tools such as patient and referring physician satisfaction surveys and analyzing historical and current practice data. Once these data are obtained, the quality improvement team can clarify service problems, identify root causes, devise solutions, and test them. Imaging is a highly competitive specialty, and facilities with quality improvement programs will ultimately prove to be the more successful groups with more efficient patient throughput and an improved bottom line.

References

1. Medical errors: focusing more on what and why, less on who. *J Oncol Pract.* 2007;3:66–70.

2. Cherry J, Seshadri S. Six Sigma: using statistics to reduce process variability and costs in radiology. *Radiol Manage.* 2000;22(6):42–45.

3. Varkey P, Reller MK, Resar RK. Basics of quality improvement in health care. *Mayo Clin Proc.* 2007;82:735–739.

4. Newmark J. From talk to action: what performance improvement is really all about. *Radiol Manage.* 2007;29(3):18–30.

5. Monopoli E. Finding Black Belt talent: the buy-make-rent dilemma. *iSixSigma.com.* Available at: http://www.isixsigma.com/library/content/c050406b.asp. Accessed March 23, 2010.

6. Benedetto AR. Six Sigma: not for the faint of heart. *Radiol Manage.* 2003;25(2)40–53.

7. Solberg LI, Kottke TE, Brekke. Quality improvement in primary care: the role of organization, collaboratives, and managed care. In: McLaughlin CP, Kaluzny AD, eds. *Continuous Quality Improvement in Health Care: Theory, Implementations, and Applications.* 3rd ed. Boston, MA: Jones and Bartlett; 2006.

8. Griffith JR, White KR. *The Well-Managed Healthcare Organization.* 5th ed. Washington, DC: AUPHA Press; 2002:261.

9. Finlayson T, Zaccardi M. Exceptional Customer Service. University of Colorado–Denver, Department of Pathology:2009. Available at: http://www.uchsc.edu/pathology/news/documents/AIDETforPathologyPhysicians-POMC-11-18-09.pdf. Accessed February 25, 2010.

10. Tunks R. *Fast Track to Quality: A 12-Month Program for Small to Mid-Sized Businesses*. New York, NY: McGraw-Hill; 1992:225.

11. Fried B, Carpenter WR. Understanding and improving team effectiveness in quality improvement. In: McLaughlin CP, Kaluzny AD, eds. *Continuous Quality Improvement in Health Care: Theory, Implementations, and Applications*. 3rd ed. Boston, MA: Jones and Bartlett; 2006.

Index

Index note: boxes are indicated by a b; *figures are indicated by an* f; *sidebars are indicated by an* s; *tables are indicated by a* t *following the page number.*